For Amanda

Acknowledgments

I have had so much support, encouragement, and hands-on assistance, and so many helpful ideas. This could take a while.

I speak from my heart: I truly could not have done this without the help of my wife Amanda DuBois. She inspired me to take on the project by pointing out, "You've been getting the inside scoop from women about their sex lives for years. Men would love to know what you know. Why not write a book about it?" Since that time she has encouraged and sometimes prodded me to keep going with my writing. She has helped me edit multiple versions. And she has consistently offered sage advice and brilliant suggestions.

My beautiful daughters, Julia and Maddy DuBois believed in me. Catharine DuBois, Rita DuBois, and Greg DuBois helped with editing and technical assistance. Bill Hoke offered suggestions, content contributions, and encouragement.

Monica Cary has been a tremendous source of support with review and comments. And she created my first "meno-party" where she invited a bunch of friends over to pepper me with questions about hot flashes, hormones, vaginal dryness, libido, moods, sex, and other women's health issues.

My therapist helped me find the confidence, focus, and clarity to go forward and complete the project.

Jayne Hulsey, Jerilyn Brusseau, and Roz Solomon have given me support, honest feedback, and ideas for promotion; and they have introduced me to other sources of help.

Pepper Schwartz provided advice based on her vast experience and expertise.

When I was planning this book, I conducted individual interviews with several men and women. I asked very personal questions so that I could test the insights and lessons about sexuality that I had acquired during my four decades of talking with thousands of women and men in my practice. Their unabashed frank sharing was invaluable.

Thank you Autumn Lerner, Alison Jacobs, Lori Mahoney, Tanya Meyers, Ki Gottberg, Jacqueline Roberts, Gwen Denombynes, Rose Pederson, Cindy Hallate, Val Lytle, Annette Abrahamson, Windy Discher, Lily Pierson, Sandra Broberg, Michael Abrahamson, Jason Cutter, Mark Thompson, Gary Blessington, Fred Rea, Bobby Marrs, and Ben Maxey.

Richard Bevan has become my catalyst for completion. His experience, advice, and hands-on assistance in editing, book design, and publishing have proven to be just what I needed to make this book a reality. His tireless support has meant everything to me.

And I must not ignore UpToDate (www.uptodate.com), an excellent online source of authoritative and reliable medical information for medical professionals. I studied their reviews on pretty much every subject that I discussed in this book. I appreciate UpToDate's cogent and comprehensive accounts of the medical information discussed here.[1]

In short, I owe much to many and I thank them all very sincerely.

Philip DuBois
Seattle, WA

---

[1] UpToDate is accessible only by subscription, so the full text of their information is not readily available. But whenever possible I have accompanied UpToDate references with articles from other sources that can be accessed directly.

CONTENTS

INTRODUCTION   1

1. THE PROBLEM—AND THE OPPORTUNITY   3
   The Realities of Sexual Intimacy   3
   Dating Your Partner   4
   Is This Book about Menopause or Sex?   5
   How the Book is Organized   6

2. WHAT IS MENOPAUSE?   9
   The Three Stages of Menopause   11
   Perimenopause   12
   True Menopause   13
   Postmenopause   15
   Birth Control during Menopause   16
   What's Next?   17

3. HOT FLASHES—IS IT HOT IN HERE?   19
   What If Men Had Hot Flashes?   19
   What Causes Hot Flashes?   20
   How Common Are Hot Flashes?   21
   Ways You Can Help Your Partner   23
   What's Next?   24

4. MR. SANDMAN, BRING ME SOME SLEEP   25
   Sleeping Problems during Menopause   25
   Some Aids for Sleep   26
   What's Next?   28

5. MEMORY LOSS: IS THIS ALZHEIMER'S?   29
   How Common Is This?   30
   What Can We Both Do about Memory Loss?   31
   What's Next?   33

6. VAGINAL PROBLEMS: OUCH, THAT HURTS   35
   The Problems of Vaginal Atrophy   36
   What's the Treatment?   37
   Nonmedical Remedies for Vaginal Atrophy   40
   What's Next?   42

7. BLADDER PROBLEMS: PUT A LITTLE TOWEL DOWN   43
   Bladder Problems in Menopause   43
   Dealing with Bladder Problems   47
   What's Next?   51

8. THE MOODY SEVEN   53
   Falling Hormone Levels   54
   Physical Changes   55
   The Empty Nest   59
   Boomerang Babies   60
   Lost Dreams   62
   Declining Intimacy   65
   Fear of Aging   68
   What's Next?   69
9. WHAT ABOUT ME, THE MAN?   71
   Testosterone   71
   The Equipment   77
   What Women Want   78
   Medical Remedies to Enhance Erections   80
   Nonmedical Remedies to Enhance Erections   83
   Think and Act Young   85
   What's Next?   88
10. SEX—LET'S KEEP THE LOVE ALIVE!   89
   Start with Good Hygiene   90
   Face Up to Falling Hormones.   91
   Be a Partner   92
   Take Care of the Romance   94
   Make Sex Dates   96
   What's Next?   99
11. PARTING THOUGHTS   101

APPENDICES

HORMONES—DOC, GIVE 'EM BACK TO HER   103
   How Estrogen Is Taken   103
   How Progestin Is Taken   105
   Bioidentical Hormones   107
   Benefits of Taking Hormones   108
   Combination Menopausal Hormones   109
   Benefits and Risks of Taking Estrogen Only   110
   Let's Review   112
   What's Next?   113
HORMONE-FREE MEDICATIONS   115
   SSRIs for Hot Flashes and Moodiness   115
   Gabapentin for Hot Flashes   116
   Clonidine Skin Patch for Hot Flashes   117
   Let's Review   117
   What's Next?   117
NATURAL REMEDIES FOR MENOPAUSAL SYMPTOMS   119
   Herbal and Nutritional Remedies   119
   Alternative Medicine and Lifestyle Alterations   121
   Let's Review   121
ABOUT THE AUTHOR   123

Introduction

I wrote this book for men whose partners are going through menopause. And I hope that women will find this information about menopause to be helpful to them as well. The book is about women and sex during the menopausal years. As a board certified obstetrician-gynecologist, I have been talking with women about their bodies and their sex lives for four decades and I have met with many of their partners along the way.

My intent is to help men understand what their partners are going through during menopause and to give them insight into how to be better partners. Typically, this translates into more intimacy—and yes, more and better sex.

In the early years of my career as an obstetrician-gynecologist, I struggled to understand how to help women and couples who complained that their sex lives were no longer satisfactory. Some women told me that they had lost the desire to make love with their partner. Others reported that their partner had stopped approaching them for sexual intimacy. An important part of their life and their relationship seemed to be over.

I talked with men who complained that their partner routinely rebuffed their sexual advances. And I talked with other men who were avoiding sex because they were having problems getting or keeping an erection.

I was at a loss. Hormones and other medications were usually not the answer. I attended medical meetings where sexual responsiveness was dissected and discussed at length. But when these meetings were concluded, I was always frustrated. I didn't come away with anything practical that I could use to help my patients.

But as I worked with women and their partners and heard their stories, I gained insights and experience. I began to notice recurring themes around sexual intimacy. I observed behaviors and attitudes that seemed to produce positive outcomes and I noticed other actions and behaviors that made things worse.

I learned a crucial lesson: hormones and techniques aren't the secret to a good sex life. Sexual intimacy naturally wanes in most relationships after the first years of "new lover passion" wear off. After this, intimacy tends to decline, along with the level of sexual activity. And as couples get older, the decline in intimacy usually continues.

But I also learned that this decline in intimacy is not inevitable. It can be revived. And intimacy is an essential ingredient for maintaining sweetness and romantic love in a relationship!

I have had a unique opportunity to hear women tell me what makes them more or less interested in sexual intimacy with their partner. I have learned disarmingly simple yet remarkably effective approaches to maintain or enhance sexual closeness. I decided that I would share these insights.

I will guide you through the powerful trifecta that has everything to do with your partner's interest and enthusiasm for sex and intimacy with you: (1) her physiologic changes during menopause, (2) life changes that you both are going through at this time of life, and (3) the powerful impact of her interactions with you, the man. Understanding these concepts will allow you to take advantage of the practical approaches that I will discuss throughout this book.

This book is not intended to replace your partner's relationship with her doctor.[2] Nor is it intended to give medical advice. Rather, it aims to give you information and guidance to help you understand the issues and take steps to strengthen your relationship with your partner.

---

[2] I use the term "doctor" as a catchall for the many types of health care providers, including medical doctors, osteopaths, nurse practitioners, and physician assistants.

CHAPTER 1

The Problem—and the Opportunity

Over the years, I've noticed several themes that have arisen repeatedly in my discussions with women about sex, intimacy, and menopause.

In this chapter I will share what I've learned from my patients about concerns and challenges that they have experienced in their relationships during menopause, and discuss some of the tactics and strategies that can help both partners—and the relationship.

THE REALITIES OF SEXUAL INTIMACY

Sexual intimacy in real life can look very different from what we read about in books, and what we see in movies and on TV. Couples should try to avoid comparing themselves unfavorably to the movie-dream-world version. The truth is that however a couple chooses to express sexual intimacy behind closed doors is just fine. We are not characters in a movie.

Sometimes—or often—sexual intimacy is swept aside by the realities of everyday life. Raising kids, taking care of the home and finances, developing and maintaining careers, and social demands push sexual intimacy into the background. Spontaneous sex tends to happen less and less often in established relationships.

And with these pressures and distractions, feelings can get hurt. Often when one partner—usually the man—approaches the other for spontaneous sex, the approachee is too busy, or tired, or preoccupied. The approacher gets hurt feelings and feels rejected and unloved. After that, the approacher protects their ego by becoming distant and less likely to make sexual overtures. Sexual intimacy becomes even less frequent.

This dwindling of sexual intimacy is common in established relationships. But that doesn't mean that sexual intimacy is not important to the partners and to the relationship. An important lesson that I have learned from my patients is that couples need sexual intimacy on a regular basis in order to maintain a nourishing and romantic relationship.

When life gets in the way of regular sexual intimacy, the relationship suffers. The warmth and tenderness wane, and couples become roommates instead of lovers. But it doesn't need to go that way. My patients have told me that they would rather have a partner and a lover than a roommate.

For reasons that we will discuss throughout this book, this diminishing sexual intimacy often comes to a head during menopause. In this book we will be exploring the actual physiologic changes, and the personal, relationship, and life style changes that may need to be dealt with during this time. Let's explore what I have learned that can restore and maintain sexual intimacy and romance around the time of menopause in a long-term relationship.

DATING YOUR PARTNER

You've probably heard about the idea of sex dates. While you may already be familiar with this notion, I think that you will find it making even more sense in the context of menopause.

After counseling women for years and listening to laments about lost romance, I have learned that the best way to restore the cycle of intimacy and romance is to put the fantasy of spontaneous sex in the back seat and put sex dates in the driver's seat.

Sex dates allow couples to plan a time when they won't be interrupted or preoccupied. Women tell me that knowing they are going to have a sex date allows them time to get into the mood. And men tell me that knowing that an intimate experience is approaching takes the pressure off and relieves them of risking rejection.

You might ask what sex dates have to do with menopause.

Well, many women tell me that their sex drive has been going downhill since their early thirties. And when they hit menopause, that hill gets steeper. Sex drive is partially dependent on a woman's hormone levels. And studies demonstrate that a woman's hormone levels begin to fall in her early thirties.

But there are many other factors that play a big part in determining the level and nature of a person's sex drive.

In this book, we will discuss how you, the man, can keep this mysterious sexual romance alive. And sex dates can be a big part of the solution. But before you jump to Chapter 10, do read the intervening chapters carefully, as they put things in the proper context for understanding the relationship changes, physiologic changes, and life changes that are taking place.

It's all about the relationship, but it sure will help if you understand how your partner's female functions work. This is why every man should have access to a good gynecologist. We have the information that you've been searching for.

To use an already well-worn—but no less valid—cliché, the biggest sex organ that a man or woman has is their brain. This is why the well-being of a couple's sex life rides so heavily on their relationship.

IS THIS BOOK ABOUT MENOPAUSE OR SEX?

These subjects are inseparable, and this book is about both. This is where the rubber hits the road. As you read on, you will learn about the tremendous changes that your partner is going through during menopause.

If your relationship is solid and supportive, you will get through this unfamiliar and potentially difficult time together and come out just fine. And your sexual relationship may well reach new heights.

I'm here to show you how you can enhance your sexual intimacy at this time of your lives by understanding your partner's journey through menopause and by being more aware of how your communication and other behaviors can affect your relationship.

I promise you won't feel as if you're going back to school as you read this. I hope and believe you will find it to be a fun and fascinating read.

HOW THE BOOK IS ORGANIZED

In Chapter 2 I'll explain what happens to your partner's body as she goes through the three stages of menopause.

In Chapters 3 through 8, I devote an entire chapter to each of the first six of the seven most common menopausal problems: Chapter 3, hot flashes; Chapter 4, sleeping problems; Chapter 5, memory loss; Chapter 6, vaginal problems; Chapter 7, bladder problems; and Chapter 8, moodiness. I'll talk about what causes these problems, how likely they are, and what can be done to make them more tolerable for your partner and ultimately for you. I'll discuss how you can be a more supportive partner during your partner's menopause. And I'll give you tips as to how you can actually enhance the sexual intimacy in your relationship.

I decided that before discussing menopausal problem number seven (sex problems), I needed to talk in detail about what we men may be going through with our bodies at the same time that our partners are going through menopause. This is what Chapter 9 is about.

In Chapter 10—drum roll—I talk all about sex.

In Chapter 11, I summarize the concepts that I offer in this book.

And in the three Appendices, I discuss in detail hormones, hormone-free medications, and nontraditional remedies for menopausal symptoms.

Throughout the book I answer typical questions that I have heard from men who have accompanied their partners to appointments during my four decades of practicing gynecology. I use these questions, and my answers, to help illustrate certain important concepts. Here's an example:

MAN QUESTION

My dad didn't help with the housework. Why should I?

DR. D's ANSWER

One thing I've heard over and over from women is that their man too often acts like a little boy around the house. *That's just not sexy!*

Women don't want to take the role of their partner's mother. They don't want to pick up after him, nor do they want to be stuck with all of the household chores like cooking, shopping, cleaning, laundry, and childcare.

Throughout this book you will find stories that illustrate some of the most important concepts. These vignettes are based on the real experiences of women and men with whom I have worked over the years. I have been amazed and inspired by the unabashed humanity that they have shared with me.

While my primary audience here is men, I hope that women will also read this book. I am confident that it contains a wealth of information that can be helpful for women.

CHAPTER 2

What Is Menopause?

MAN QUESTION

What does my partner's menopause have to do with me anyway?

DR. D'S ANSWER

Your partner's menopause has pretty much everything to do with you. Many of my patients have told me that their mood, their sex drive, their ability to have comfortable sex, and their health in general is impacted when they are going through menopause.

Understanding these issues will help you to be a supportive partner during your partner's menopause. And you will learn how you can parlay this knowledge to make your sexual relationship way better than it may have been for years.

ANOTHER MAN QUESTION

Doc, my partner says that she thinks she's going through menopause. I've heard of it, of course, but I really have no clue. What is it?

DR. D'S ANSWER

Menopause is the time in a woman's life when:

- Her ovaries stop producing the hormones estrogen and progesterone.
- Her ovaries stop releasing eggs.
- Her periods become irregular and eventually stop.

YET ANOTHER MAN QUESTION

What is estrogen?

DR. D'S ANSWER

Estrogen is the primary female hormone. This hormone is produced every day of the month from the time of puberty until menopause.

Sex, Intimacy, and Menopause

Here's what estrogen does prior to menopause.

- Every month, estrogen thickens your partner's endometrium (uterine lining) to prepare it for supporting a pregnancy. If no pregnancy occurs that cycle, the endometrium is shed. This is her period.
- Estrogen keeps your partner's vagina moist, elastic, and tough. This allows her to have comfortable sex.
- Estrogen supports development and maintenance of your partner's breasts, and it enhances her sex drive.

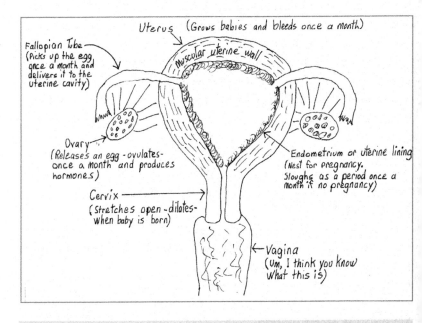

MAN QUESTION

What is progesterone?

DR. D'S ANSWER

Progesterone is the other female hormone.

Prior to menopause, your partner ovulates (releases an egg from one of her ovaries) every month. After she ovulates, that ovary begins to produce progesterone.

Here's what progesterone does prior to menopause:

- After ovulation, progesterone stimulates your partner's uterine lining to thicken, produce mucous, and develop an enhanced blood supply. This prepares a "nest" for the fertilized egg in case a pregnancy has occurred that cycle.
- If the egg was not fertilized with sperm (no pregnancy), the egg will disintegrate and progesterone production will cease after about fourteen days.
- Progesterone is necessary to maintain your partner's uterine lining. Without it the lining breaks down and is shed as her period.

All women go through menopause. In 90 percent of women, these changes take place sometime between ages of forty-five and fifty-five.

THE THREE STAGES OF MENOPAUSE

Menopause or "change of life" occurs in three stages. I'll tell you what these stages are, and then I'll describe them in detail.

- **Perimenopause** is the first stage and consists of the preliminary changes that your partner goes through over a period of two to five years prior to the time that her periods stop altogether.
- **True menopause**[3] is the second stage. This is the time when your partner's periods have stopped for good, and she has had no vaginal bleeding for one full year.
- **Postmenopause** is the third stage, and is simply the state that your partner is in for the rest of her life from the time that she has completed true menopause. And by the way, there is a lot more good living and good sex for both of you during postmenopause.

Except for vaginal bleeding patterns, the possible symptoms are the same in each of the three stages of menopause. But the severity of the

---

[3] To avoid confusion, I use the term "true menopause" to indicate the time when a woman's periods have stopped for good. And I use the term "menopause" to describe all three stages.

symptoms may vary with each stage and they will vary with each woman. Here they are:

- Hot flashes with sweat attacks
- Problems with sleeping and night sweats
- Forgetfulness
- Vaginal problems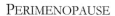
- Bladder problems
- Moodiness
- Decreased sex drive

PERIMENOPAUSE

During the two to five years prior to your partner's last period she will go through a preliminary stage called perimenopause.

This is the time when her ovaries are gradually losing their capacity to produce adequate amounts of the female hormones, estrogen and progesterone. Her ovaries will still be working, but not at full capacity.

Vaginal Bleeding in Perimenopause

Women in their forties often come to see me with concerns about irregular vaginal bleeding. Most have been having regular periods up to this point. But now they are feeling the same frustration with irregular periods that they felt when they were in their teens.

They don't know when they're going to bleed or for how long. Some women with irregular bleeding are finding that they have to go back to wearing a light-day pad every day to protect themselves from unexpected bleeding onto their clothes.

Here's how your partner's periods may change during perimenopause. It would be normal for her periods to be shorter, lighter, or farther apart than they were when she was in her thirties. Her ovaries are producing less estrogen, so her uterine lining is not stimulated to build up as thick. The result is less uterine lining to slough, bleed, and be expelled.

But if she has periods that are longer, heavier, or closer together, that's not normal. In this case she should see her doctor for testing.

MAN QUESTION

Didn't you say that we would be talking about sex?

DR. D'S ANSWER

We'll be talking about sex throughout this book, and Chapter 10 will be devoted entirely to sex.

The pages that don't directly reference sex will help you better understand how your partner's body works. Understanding what your partner is going through will enrich your relationship. And remember, sex is all about the relationship.

TRUE MENOPAUSE

The definition of true menopause is twelve months of no vaginal bleeding in a woman over age forty. As your partner is approaching true menopause, she may go a few months without a period, and then have one or two or three periods, and then go a few more months without bleeding. But your partner will not be in true menopause until she has gone a full year with no bleeding.

MAN QUESTION

What should I do if my partner's periods are heavier or longer?

DR. D'S ANSWER

If your partner's periods are heavier or longer, or if she bleeds more than once a month, encourage her to see her doctor. An abnormal bleeding pattern could be an indication of polyps or a precancerous growth of her uterine lining—or even cancer. The source of the abnormal bleeding can be treated as long as it is not ignored.

Some women ignore abnormal bleeding patterns because they're afraid that they might get bad news when they see their doctor. Offer to accompany your partner when she goes to see her doctor. But if you do go with her, be careful not to take over the visit. Think of yourself as her support person, not her manager.

And do lend a sympathetic ear when your partner expresses frustration with the unpredictable bleeding.

MAN QUESTION

Should my partner be tested for menopause?

DR. D'S ANSWER

Not really. See the box below.

Menopause and testing

Currently the best test for menopause is to measure a blood sample for elevated levels of follicle-stimulating hormone (FSH). A woman's pituitary gland (the body's hormone control center located at the base of the brain—see drawing on page 21) releases FSH whenever her estrogen level is too low. FSH's job is to stimulate her ovaries to produce adequate amounts of estrogen.

As menopause approaches, a woman's ovaries lose their capacity to produce adequate amounts of estrogen even when stimulated. To compensate, her pituitary gland releases more and more FSH to stimulate her ovaries to keep up. The resulting elevated FSH levels that may be detected in a blood sample during any of the three stages of menopause would be an indication of menopause.

But the test is not reliable. FSH is not consistently elevated during any stage of menopause; it fluctuates up and down. A woman going through menopause may have a normal FSH one moment and an elevated FSH the next.

Testing women forty years and older for menopause is usually a waste of time and money. Your partner might as well wring the sweat from her shirt into a beaker and have her doctor test that. If your partner is in her forties or early fifties and is experiencing hot flashes and other menopausal symptoms, she is most likely entering menopause.

On the other hand, if your partner has these symptoms prior to age forty, she should be tested.

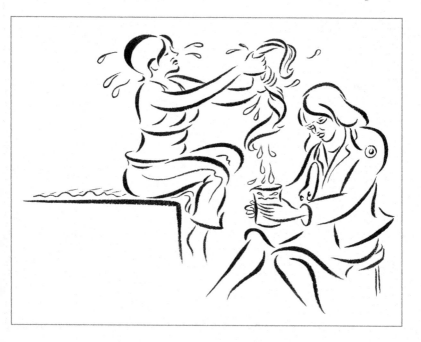

POSTMENOPAUSE

Postmenopause, as the term implies, is simply the phase of menopause that continues during the remainder of your partner's life after she has completed true menopause. All the symptoms described at the beginning of this chapter may continue to occur during this time. Remedies for menopausal symptoms are discussed in detail in Appendices 1, 2, and 3.

It's possible that your partner may experience vaginal bleeding after menopause. Postmenopausal bleeding (PMB) is any vaginal bleeding (even a brown, pink, or red discharge) that happens more than a year after a woman's last period.

PMB is not normal. In fact, bleeding that happens more than just six months after a woman's last period may need to be evaluated. Cancer of the uterine lining must be ruled out. Cancer, though not likely, is the cause of PMB 5 to 10 percent of the time.

MAN QUESTION

So Doc, what do you recommend if my partner has any abnormal bleeding?

DR. D'S ANSWER

Encourage your partner to see her doctor if she has any bleeding at all after menopause.

ANOTHER MAN QUESTION

Can my partner get pregnant during any of the stages of menopause?

DR. D'S ANSWER

Great question!

Pregnancy is not likely during menopause, but it is possible. During your partner's perimenopausal years (early to mid forties) her fertility (ability to get pregnant naturally) will decline rapidly. See the next section.

BIRTH CONTROL DURING MENOPAUSE

When a woman gets into her forties, her ovaries begin to go dormant. They actually shrink in size and produce less estrogen and progesterone. And the remaining eggs will gradually disintegrate. Less than two-thirds of women in their early forties are able to get pregnant naturally.[4] After age forty-five, most women (92 percent) are not fertile.[5,6] In my entire career, I have not seen a woman over age forty-five get pregnant and carry that pregnancy to a live birth unless she has had assistance from drugs or surgery. Pregnancy can happen, but it's rare.

The safest approach to prevent pregnancy would be for your partner to wait until she is past age fifty and has gone through true

---

[4] Menken, Trussell, and Larsen, "Age and Infertility" (*Science*, Vol. 233, No. 4771, 1986, pp. 1389-94)

[5] Tietze, "Reproductive Span and Rate of Reproduction among Hutterite Women" (*Fertility and Sterility*, Vol. 8, No. 89, 1957, pp. 89-97)

[6] Laufer, Simon, Samueloff, Yaffe, Milwidsky, and Gielchinsky, "Successful Spontaneous Pregnancies in Women Older Than 45 Years (*Fertility and Sterility*, Vol. 81, No. 5, 2004, pp. 1328-32)

menopause (one year with no periods) before she stops using birth control.

But if your partner is on birth control pills, she will probably continue having periods even if her body is in menopause. This is because the hormones in the pill stimulate her uterine lining to build up and slough even if her ovaries are no longer able to make their own hormones. And the hormones in the pill will probably prevent hot flashes and other menopausal symptoms.

If your partner is still on the pill when she reaches fifty, she should talk to her doctor. There are increased risks associated with birth control pill use by this age.

WHAT'S NEXT?

Chapters 3 through 8 are about the symptoms of menopause. The seventh symptom, lower sex drive, is Chapter 10. Guys, this is eye-opening information. I'm going to help you to understand the changes that have been distressing your partner and perhaps troubling you. I venture to say that this will be like a drink of the cool water of understanding while in the desert of bewildering menopausal symptoms.

We'll talk about hot flashes in the next chapter. What are they? How likely are they? What causes them? How are they like an HVAC system in a building? How might they impact you and your partner's sex life? And how can you support your partner as she deals with them?

CHAPTER 3

Hot Flashes—Is It Hot in Here?

MAN QUESTION

I think that my partner is having hot flashes. She gets really hot and sweaty at times. There's not much that can be done about hot flashes, is there?

DR. D.'S ANSWER

Well, actually there is a lot that can be done. Just understanding the symptoms of menopause goes a long way. This will allow you to be supportive of your partner and will make it easier for you to go through menopause with her—rather than standing on the sideline confused and helpless. And there are many remedies for hot flashes that I'll tell you about.

So let's dive in here and see what we can learn about hot flashes, the harbinger symptom of menopause.

WHAT IF MEN HAD HOT FLASHES?

Imagine that you, a man, are at work or hanging out with your friends. Out of the blue you get a hot feeling in your face and upper chest. The intense heat spreads to the rest of your body.

Your skin stays cool. And after what seems like an eternity, the hot feeling inside you starts to let up. But now your skin turns red and hot and you start to sweat.

Then you feel light headed and there's a pounding inside your chest. You think that you're having a heart attack. You look around for a place to drop.

You don't want anybody to think that you're not tough, so you try to act as if everything is normal. You wonder if anyone notices that something's happening to you. When you get concerned looks from your friends, you shrug, "I think I must be coming down with a bug."

You feel better in a few minutes, but now you're soaking wet. You fake it through this one. But as the weeks go by these weird attacks come more and more often, usually with no warning.

At times your face, or legs, or feet get so hot that you have to use a damp cloth to cool them off. You've learned to bring a change of clothes wherever you go because you usually sweat profusely when you have these heat attacks. And you wear clothes in layers so that you can take the outer layers off and put them back on as you get hot and cold during these spells.

And lately you're been having trouble sleeping. You wake up at night soaking with sweat. You throw off the covers. Then you get cold and start to shiver, so you pull the covers back on. But now the sheets are wet from your sweat.

You can't get back to sleep unless you change the sheets. This wakes up your partner. At first she tries to be sympathetic, but she's getting cranky. "Are you getting old?" she asks.

WHAT CAUSES HOT FLASHES?

Hot flashes are caused by the brain's response to low estrogen levels. Your partner's pituitary gland, located at the base of the brain, detects the low estrogen levels and sends out an ovarian stimulating hormone called follicle-stimulating hormone (FSH) to drive her ovaries harder to do what they no longer can do (produce adequate amounts of estrogen).

The thermoregulatory center of your partner's brain, her thermostat, which sits just next door to her pituitary gland, is disturbed by the increased activity of her pituitary as it produces extra FSH.

Your partner's thermoregulatory center responds to this disturbance by narrowing its thermoneutral zone. It begins to function like a faulty heating/air conditioning system that alternately triggers back and forth between heat and A/C because the range for normal temperature fluctuations is too narrow.

The result is that your partner's body is too often either cooling itself by dilating the blood vessels of her skin (making her feel hot and flushed) and sweating for the evaporative cooling.

Or it's reheating itself by shivering to produce more heat from her skeletal muscle contractions. Women often feel hot and cold at the same time when this happens.

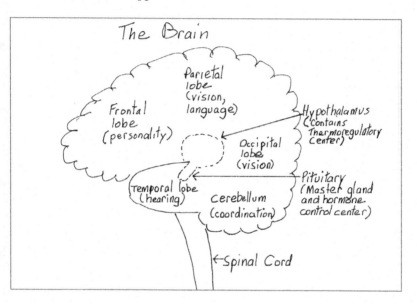

HOW COMMON ARE HOT FLASHES?

- About 75 percent of women experience hot flashes while they are going through menopause.[7]
- More than 40 percent of women have hot flashes during perimenopause (the two to five years before periods stop).
- More than 55 percent of women begin hot flashes at true menopause (the time that their periods stop for good).[8]

---

[7] Santen, Loprinzi, and Casper, "Menopausal Hot Flashes" (Jan 20, 2015, UpToDate, www.uptodate.com)

[8] National Institutes of Health State-of-the-Science Conference statement, "Management of Menopause–Related Symptoms" (*Annals of Internal Medicine,* Vol. 142, 2005, p. 1003)

- Hot flashes persist for more than a year in 80 percent of menopausal women.
- Hot flashes persist past age sixty in about 14 percent of women.[9] And they will continue past age seventy in 9 percent of women.
- Hot flashes occur anywhere from once a day to as often as more than once an hour.

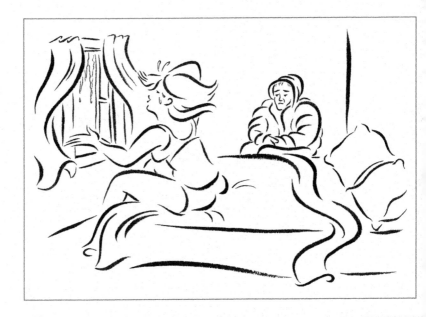

MAN QUESTION

Great! So this thermoregulatory breakdown could go on for several years? Can you give me some hope to go on?

DR. D'S ANSWER

Don't despair. There are lots of remedies. These are discussed in detail in Appendices 1, 2, and 3. Let's talk about how *you* can help.

---

[9] Rödström, Bengtsson, Lissner, Milsom, Sundh, and Björkelund, "A Longitudinal Study of the Treatment of Hot Flushes, the Population Study of Women in Gothenburg during a Quarter of a Century" (*Menopause*, Vol. 9., No. 3, 2002, pp. 156-61)

WAYS YOU CAN HELP YOUR PARTNER

To assist your partner as she deals with hot flashes, the most important thing is for you to be a good sport.

- Don't tease her or act impatient or disinterested when she asks, "Is it hot in here?"
- Let her know that you are reading about what she's going through, and that you will do whatever you can to help her be more comfortable.
- If you buy her clothes, don't get her a pullover or turtleneck sweater. And don't even think of getting her anything wool or cashmere. Sweaters and jackets that zip in front are easier to take off and put back on.
- You could get your partner a beautiful handheld fan and one of those tiny battery powered fans.
- Even better, you could install air conditioning.
- Let her control the heat in the house and in the car.
- Dress in layers yourself so that you can be comfortable as she adjusts the heat up and down. And she will, I promise.

I have often shared a glass of wine and watched the news with my wife in the winter with the heat turned off and a window or two opened. She'll be in a tank top and I'll be in fleece.

And I still wear socks, sweatpants, and a hooded sweatshirt when we go to bed with the windows open and the fan on.

MAN QUESTION

This doesn't sound very sexy for my partner to be sweating and me freezing. I don't want our sex life to be over. Is it?

DR. D'S ANSWER

Your sex life will probably change. Your partner's sex drive may diminish because of her discomfort from hot flashes, the drop in her estrogen levels, and several other factors that are discussed throughout this book and detailed in Chapter 10.

But your sex life can be as good or better when you understand what's happening and when the two of you learn to adjust to the changes. As we go along, we will talk a lot about how you, the man, can help keep the love alive.

WHAT'S NEXT?

In the next chapter we talk about sleep disturbances in menopause. Many women complain to me of difficulty sleeping while going through the three stages of menopause. There are many factors that contribute to this problem. Fortunately there are lots of ways to improve it.

Personally, I find it to be frustrating when my wife has trouble sleeping. I do whatever I can to make it easier for her. I'd like to fix this problem, but there's only so much that I can do. But she does appreciate my concern and efforts.

As the man, your response to your partner's sleeplessness can make a difference.

CHAPTER 4

Mr. Sandman, Bring Me Some Sleep

Doc, my partner used to sleep like a rock. Now, not so much. Anything I can do about this?

There certainly is. And thanks for the great question. Let's talk about it.

SLEEPING PROBLEMS DURING MENOPAUSE

Hot flashes typically occur more commonly at night, and they are notorious for disturbing sleep. But menopausal women who are not having hot flashes may also have problems sleeping.

Women tell me that they sweat so heavily at night that they have to get up and change their pajamas and the sheets. They complain that even tiny light sources bother them. And some say they have racing thoughts.

About 36 percent of menopausal women have sleeping problems during perimenopause. These disturbances increase to about 42 percent as women approach true menopause.[10] Sleep disturbance is more likely during the first four hours of the night.

There are a variety of strategies that can assist in improving sleep. Let's first look at strategies that don't involve medication or supplements.

- Lower the temperature in the bedroom. This can help a lot. So guys, put on your sweatshirt, sweatpants, and long johns, and let your partner play freeze-out to her heart's content.
- Pretend that you're on a camping trip. Don't complain if she

---

[10] Casper, "Clinical Manifestations and Diagnosis of Menopause" (Feb 4, 2014, UpToDate, www.uptodate.com)

throws the blankets off and back on during the night. [11]

- Run a fan all night. My patients have told me that this helps them stay cool and dry, and the sound of the fan helps them to sleep. Get a nice stainless steel fan instead of a cheap plastic one.
- Keep the lights down. Light sources—even tiny ones—bother some women. Cover the lights on phones, computers, and smoke detectors. Ask your partner if she would like blackout shades.
- If all else fails, try some of the sleep aids discussed in the next section, or the menopausal remedies described in the Appendices.

One more idea: I read to my wife every night. This puts her right to sleep. We are careful to choose books that are inspiring and uplifting. We look for books that will quiet our minds. Some of our favorites are:

- *Spiritual Liberation* by Michael Bernard Beckwith
- *The Spontaneous Fulfillment of Desire* by Deepak Chopra
- *There's a Spiritual Solution to Every Problem* by Wayne W. Dyer
- *The Four Agreements* by Don Miguel Ruiz

SOME AIDS FOR SLEEP

Melatonin is a hormone produced by the pineal gland in the brain. It is known to promote sleep.[12] Natural production of melatonin declines gradually after age forty in both sexes. This decline in melatonin production is thought to contribute to sleep problems in older women and men. Sleep patterns often improve with melatonin supplementation.

- Dose: If your doctor approves, the recommended dose is 0.3 mg at bedtime. This can be repeated in fifteen to thirty minutes if needed. Melatonin can be purchased over the counter at health food stores. *Most often the over-the-counter dose is at least ten times higher than 0.3 mg. You may need to purchase melatonin in liquid form and use a dropper to deliver the proper dose.*

---

[11] Freedman and Roehrs, "Effects of REM Sleep and Ambient Temperature on Hot Flash-Induced Sleep Disturbance" (*Menopause*, Vol. 13, No. 4, 2006, pp. 576–83)

[12] Wurtman, "Physiology and Available Preparations of Melatonin" (Apr 15, 2015, UpToDate, www.uptodate.com)

- Good to know: Your partner should check with her doctor to confirm that it is safe for her to take melatonin. Daytime sleepiness and hangovers are sometimes seen as side effects, especially if too high a dose is taken.
- Caution 1: Worsening of sleep patterns is sometimes a problem after prolonged use of melatonin. If the melatonin has been working but then stops working, your partner should stop it for a couple weeks and then restart.
- Caution 2: Women with epilepsy (seizure disorder) and women taking anticoagulants (blood thinners) should discuss with their doctor whether melatonin is a good idea.

Valerian root is an herbal remedy that is commonly used for insomnia.
- Good to know: Clinical studies have not confirmed Valerian root to be effective.
- Caution 1: Liver damage is a risk with its use.[13]
- Caution 2: Use only if advised by your doctor.

Prescription sleeping pills may be an option. If your partner is still sleepless in Seattle (or wherever), she may want to consider these. Offer to pick them up for her at the pharmacy.

Caution: sleeping pills can be habituating, so it would be best if they are not taken every night. That said, don't watchdog your partner's use of them.

MAN QUESTION
Since my partner is lying there awake, does that mean that we will be having more sex?

---

[13] Bonnet and Arand, "Treatment of Insomnia" (Sept 2, 2014, UpToDate, www.uptodate.com)

DR. D'S ANSWER

Uh, you are kidding, right? I'm sure that you are aware that when she is lying there awake and throwing off the covers, it's not because she's thinking about sex. It is probably because she is soaked with sweat and miserable. This would not be a good time to make your move.

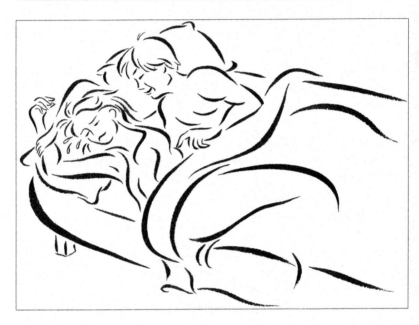

Communicating that you understand and care about what your partner is going through will go a long way toward enriching your relationship. This will open channels of communication and provide opportunities to plan for sex dates.

WHAT'S NEXT?

Women in their forties and beyond often complain of forgetfulness. In the next chapter we'll talk about the causes and prevalence of memory loss, and what can be done about it.

CHAPTER 5

Memory Loss: Is This Alzheimer's?

EILEEN'S STORY

Eileen is a forty-six-year-old former stay-at-home mom. Her three kids are no longer living at home and she now works as a legal assistant.

"Doctor, I'm starting to notice some forgetfulness. Sometimes I can't remember names of familiar people or places that I previously knew. Is this from menopause? Am I getting Alzheimer's?"

I do a neurologic exam. I find no suggestion of an undiagnosed stroke or brain damage from any other cause. Then we talk.

"Many studies have looked at memory problems in women past age forty," I explain. "It turns out that mild forgetfulness is more likely a function of age and less likely to be caused by hormonal status or early Alzheimer's. And most people with mild forgetfulness function perfectly normally.[14,15] That said, I have had some women tell me that their memory improved when they took hormones."

After we discuss the pros and cons of estrogen use, Eileen says, "No thanks." We then go over the various strategies that she can use to maintain or even improve mental prowess without taking medication. Eileen is motivated to avoid hormones and decides to take this approach.

Let's look further into memory and brain function in menopausal women. First a frequently-asked question.

---

[14] Petersen, Smith, Kokmen, Ivnik, and Tangalos, "Memory Function in Normal Aging" (*Neurology*, Vol. 42, No. 2, p. 396)
[15] Shadlen and Larson, "Evaluation of Cognitive Impairment and Dementia" (Feb 12, 2014, UpToDate, www.uptodate.com)

MAN QUESTION
Is all memory loss from Alzheimer's?
DR. D.'S ANSWER
Oh hell no!

Alzheimer's is characterized by a gradual but progressive deterioration of a person's mental capacities.

The condition generally starts with a person having increasingly severe difficulty remembering events, handling complex tasks such as paying bills, coping with unexpected events, getting lost in familiar places, and worsening difficulty finding words while talking.

Mild memory changes, on the other hand, remain fairly stable and they don't progress, or only minimally progress.[16] They remain mild and do not significantly affect daily function.[17]

HOW COMMON IS THIS?
Alzheimer's and other types of dementia (severe mental deterioration) are seen in about 5 percent of women past age sixty, and about 12 percent of women past age seventy-five.

But mild memory change is pretty much universal. It is usually first noticeable around age fifty.

MAN QUESTION
Psst! Don't tell anybody. But my memory isn't as good as it used to be either. What's that all about?
DR. D'S ANSWER
I applaud your honesty! Get this: Statistical evidence is clear that most men notice mild memory loss at about the same age that their partner does. In fact, after age seventy, we men are more likely to suffer memory

---

[16] U.S. Department of Health and Human Services Agency for Health Care Policy and Research. Clinical Practice Guidelines, Number 19. 1996.
[17] Recognition and Initial Assessment of Alzheimer's Disease and Related Dementias. AHCPR Publication No. 97-0702. Nov 1996.

loss than are women.[18] But we men don't have a life-change signpost like menopause to blame it on. So we call our memory lapses "senior moments" or "brain farts."

FOLLOW-UP MAN QUESTION

Oh boy! What can we do about the memory loss? I hope that I can remember what you tell me.

DR. D's ANSWER

Lifestyle habits can have a big impact on brain health. See below for things you can do to deal with normal mild forgetfulness.

WHAT CAN WE BOTH DO ABOUT MEMORY LOSS?

- Get plenty of exercise. This promotes improved blood flow to your brain.

- Eat a healthy diet with lots of greens and fiber. This discourages cerebral arteriosclerosis (clogged arteries to your brain) and promotes normal blood sugar levels. Avoid processed foods.

- Supplement your diet with vitamins B12[19] and D3,[20] if your doctor approves.

- Exercise your brain. Active learning keeps our brains healthy: learn a language; subscribe to a journal; get your partner a magazine on a subject in which she has expressed interest; learn a musical instrument; take dancing lessons; enroll in courses online or at the local community college.

---

[18] Petersen, Roberts, Knopman, Geda, Cha, Pankratz, Boeve, Tangalos, Ivnik, and Rocca, "Prevalence of Mild Cognitive Impairment Is Higher in Men. The Mayo Clinc Study of Aging" (*Neurology*, Vol. 75, No. 10, 2010, pp. 889–97)

[19] Deficiencies of vitamin B12 are well known to cause problems with coordination and memory. Dissolve 500 mcg of vitamin B12 under your tongue every other day. Women and men past age forty are less likely to absorb B12 adequately from their diet because of lowered production of stomach acid at this age. The sublingual (under the tongue) absorption bypasses the stomach.

[20] Take 500 to 1000 IU of vitamin D3 every other day. The statistics are less clear, but vitamin D3 deficiency may be the cause of neuropsychiatric (nervous system and mental) problems.

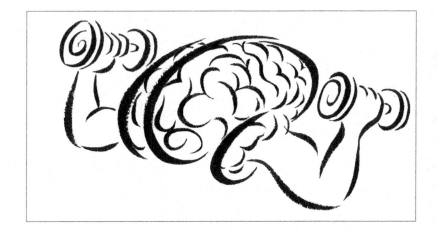

- Take 81 mg of aspirin daily if your doctor approves. Low doses of aspirin may promote good blood flow to your brain.[21]
- Maintain a healthy weight. This lowers the risk of arteriosclerosis, hypertension (high blood pressure), and diabetes—conditions that can reduce blood flow to the brain.
- Avoid cigarettes, recreational drugs, and excess alcohol. Cigarettes reduce blood flow to your brain. Drugs and alcohol impair brain function.
- Meditate or pray daily. This reduces stress, which can impair concentration and memory.
- Reassure each other that forgetfulness is no big deal, and it doesn't mean you are losing your mind or developing Alzheimer's. Laugh about it, but don't tease or mock.
- Be kind to each other. At this time in life especially, you should be thoughtful about what you say to each other, and how you say it. Instead of saying, "You're getting forgetful," say, "I do that too. It'll come to you." Don't say: "You're getting old," or "You're having a senior moment," say, "You'll think of it in a minute."

---

[21] If while taking aspirin you notice an increased tendency to bruise or prolonged bleeding when you get cut, decrease the aspirin to every other day.

- A great book that may help is *Super Brain: Unleashing the Explosive Power of Your Mind to Maximize Health, Happiness, and Spiritual Well-Being* by Rudolph E. Tanzi and Deepak Chopra.

MAN QUESTION

That's all fine and good. But what does it have to do with sex?

DR. D'S ANSWER

Oh yeah, this book is supposed to be about sex. Actually, this is.

It's not sexy to criticize or tease your partner about being forgetful. And the better you understand what your partner is going through during her menopausal changes, the better your interactions with her will be. This opens up more opportunities for sexual intimacy.

WHAT'S NEXT?

In the next chapter, we'll talk about vaginal problems that can occur during menopause. These problems can get in the way of comfortable sex. But the good news is that they don't have to.

CHAPTER 6

Vaginal Problems: Ouch, That Hurts

JEN'S DILEMMA

Jen, who has just turned fifty, comes to see me for sex problems. Jen had previously shared with me that she and her husband had an active and gratifying sex life together.

Today Jen is more somber than her usual self. I ask her what's going on.

"Doctor, in the last few months Dave and I have pretty much stopped having sex."

"Tell me more," I say.

"Well it seems that I've gotten a lot more dry down there. When Dave tries to put his penis in me, it won't go in and it hurts."

"Have you tried using lubricants like K-Y Jelly or Astroglide?"

Jen blushes. "At first Dave tried to get me wet with his tongue. That helped a little but not enough. Then we got some K-Y Jelly. With the K-Y, Dave was able to get his penis into me just fine but it hurt some. And it seems to be hurting more each time that we try. We haven't had sex for a few weeks now because Dave is afraid of hurting me. Frankly I'm relieved that he has backed off."

I examine Jen and find that her vagina is smooth, pale, and dry. The medical term for this condition is atrophic vaginitis, or vaginal atrophy.[22] It results from the low estrogen levels that occur in menopause.

After the exam, I sit with Jen and explain the problem. Even though the K-Y provides lubrication, sex is painful because her vagina has lost its elasticity as a result of the low estrogen levels in her body. When Dave stretches her unstretchable vagina with his penis, it hurts.

Vaginal estrogen is the most effective remedy for vaginal atrophy. And fortunately women will usually tolerate it well. When low doses of estrogen are placed directly into the vagina, there is minimal absorption into the rest

---

[22] Sobel, "Causes of Vaginitis" (*New England Journal of Medicine*, Vol. 337, 1997, p. 1896)

> of the body. Estrogen's local effect enables the vagina to regain its normal thickness, blood flow, elasticity, and moisture.
>
> After discussing the options, Jen decides to give vaginal estrogen a try.

Let's look further into menopausal vaginal dryness and vaginal atrophy.

Before menopause, a woman's vagina is deep pink, moist, and wrinkled. The deep pink coloration is the result of good capillary blood flow. The good blood flow provides the moisture that serves as a natural lubricant for intercourse. The wrinkles allow for stretching of the vagina during sex and childbirth.

Vaginal dryness becomes more prevalent as a woman gets deeper into menopause.

- About 20 percent of women complain of vaginal dryness as they approach true menopause.
- Almost half of women have vaginal dryness within three years postmenopause.[23]

THE PROBLEMS OF VAGINAL ATROPHY

With the low estrogen levels in menopause there is decreased blood flow to your partner's vaginal wall. As a result your partner's vagina may become thin, dry, fragile, less elastic, or even too narrow for sex. Intercourse can be difficult and painful since the nerve endings are more exposed. And you have to push harder with your penis because of the decreased elasticity and lack of natural lubrication. Ouch!

There may be a watery yellow discharge with an odor. As the vaginal wall thins from low estrogen levels, it may ooze serum from the capillary bed just beneath its surface and it may lose its ability to suppress the growth of odor producing bacteria. An odorous discharge can result.

Low estrogen levels can also cause decreased blood flow to the vulva (clitoris and vaginal lips). Your partner may experience decreased

---

[23] Bachmann and Santen "Clinical Manifestations and Diagnosis of Vaginal Atrophy" (Jun 3, 2015, UpToDate, www.uptodate.com)

sensation during sex play. With the vaginal thinning, the nerve endings are more exposed. But the predominant nerve fibers now are pain receptors. The pleasure receptors are no longer dominant. So your partner may experience less—or no—pleasure with sex.

A woman with vaginal atrophy is often less interested in intercourse because of the tenderness and decreased sensation that result from the dryness and thinning of her vaginal wall. And the lowered estrogen levels may also contribute to her lowered sex drive.

WHAT'S THE TREATMENT?
Vaginal atrophy is usually easy to treat. There are two medical remedies available: vaginal estrogen and ospemifene. There are also nonmedical remedies.

Vaginal Estrogen
Your partner can replace the estrogen that's missing in her vagina. Vaginal estrogen, which must be prescribed by her doctor, comes in the forms of creams, tablets, or soft Silastic vaginal rings.

- Creams and tablets: These are inserted using an applicator, a hollow tube loaded with the estrogen cream or tablet. Your partner will insert the applicator up to the top of her vagina and push out the cream or tablet with the plunger two or three nights a week.
- The Silastic ring is a soft flexible ring that your partner places into her vagina and leaves there. Estrogen gradually leeches out of the ring over three months, at which time she will replace it.

The vaginal ring can be left in place during intercourse. Most women don't feel it once it is in place. And most men don't feel the ring during intercourse. If either of you prefer, it can be removed prior to intercourse and replaced afterwards.

MAN QUESTION
What about the risks of estrogen?
DR. D'S ANSWER
The nice thing about vaginal estrogen is that, when used at a dose intended for vaginal atrophy, it is absorbed only into your partner's vaginal wall and surrounding tissues. The amount of estrogen that might be absorbed into the rest of her body is minimal. Estrogen levels in the blood of a woman using vaginal estrogen at a dose intended for atrophic vaginitis will remain in the menopausal range.[24]

ANOTHER MAN QUESTION
That's good to hear. But I wonder if getting that estrogen on me is going to shrink my penis.
DR. D'S ANSWER
Interesting question. The answer is no. I have never heard or read of any affects on a man from exposure of his penis or tongue to estrogen.

Vaginal estrogen should have no effect on the rest of a woman's body. That said, women with breast cancer and other estrogen-sensitive tumors might be advised by their doctor to stay off all forms of estrogen, even vaginal.

The good news is that after your partner has been using vaginal estrogen for a couple of months, her vagina should be back to its usual tough, moist, elastic self. *She needs to keep using the estrogen though. If she stops using it, the dryness and tenderness with sex will probably come back.*

Ospemifene
Ospemifene, usually known by its brand name Osphena, is a recently released selective estrogen receptor modulator (SERM). Drugs in the SERM class act like estrogen in certain parts of a woman's body and act

---

[24] Weisberg, Ayton, Darling, Farrell, Murkies, O'Neill, Kirkegard, and Fraser, "Endometrial and Vaginal Effects of Low-dose Estradiol Delivered by Vaginal Ring or Vaginal Tablet" (*Climactric*, Vol. 8, No. 1, 2005, pp. 83–92)

like an estrogen antagonist in other parts. Osphena acts like estrogen in a woman's vagina.

Does it work? In one trial, more than 50 percent of women taking ospemifene for dyspareunia (painful sex) due to vaginal atrophy reported a greater than 50 percent improvement.

How does ospemifene affect other parts of a woman's body? There appears to be no estrogen effect on the breasts while taking it. No soreness or enlargement and no increased risk of breast cancer have been demonstrated so far.

Women taking ospemifene may have some thickening of their endometrium (uterine lining). But, thus far, no uterine cancers or precancerous changes have been seen. [25, 26]

Hot flashes appear to be twice as likely in women taking ospemifene. This may be an important consideration for your partner.

As is true with estrogen itself, there is an increased risk of thromboembolism (blood clots forming in the legs and traveling to the lungs or brain) with drugs in the SERM class. So far, though, this rare complication has not been seen with ospemifene.

Ospemifene has a beneficial estrogen-like effect on bones. It appears to make them stronger, thereby reducing the risk of osteoporosis and fractures. [27]

How is it taken? Ospemifene is a tablet that must be taken once a day. This is a prescription drug, so your partner will need to see her doctor to determine whether this drug might be a good remedy for her vaginal dryness or vaginal atrophy.

[25] Bachmann and Santen, "Treatment of Vaginal Atrophy" (Apr 4, 2014, UpToDate, www.uptodate.com)

[26] Bachmann, Komi, and Ospemifene Study Group, "Ospemifene Effectively Treats Vulvovaginal Atrophy in Postmenopausal Women: Results from a Pivotal Phase 3 Study" (*Menopause*, Vol. 17, No. 3, 2010, pp. 480–6)

[27] Komi, Heikkinen, Rutanen, Halonen, Lammintausta, and Ylikorkala, "Effects of Ospemifene, a Novel SERM, on Biochemical Markers of Bone Turnover in Healthy Postmenopausal Women" (*Gynecological Endocrinology*, Vol. 18, No. 3, 2004, pp. 152–8)

MAN QUESTION

How do I fit in here (no pun intended)?

DR. D'S ANSWER

Encourage your partner to talk to her provider about getting started on vaginal estrogen. It works quite well and is very safe for most women when used at doses intended just for the vaginal effect.

If your partner can't or doesn't want to put estrogen into her vagina, she may want to talk with her doctor about taking ospemifene.

FOLLOW-UP MAN QUESTION

What if she doesn't want to use either vaginal estrogen or ospe—whatever?

DR. D'S ANSWER

There are nonmedical approaches that can improve vaginal dryness and tenderness with intercourse. They are less helpful when the condition is more severe, but they work well for some women. See the next section for some examples.

NONMEDICAL REMEDIES FOR VAGINAL ATROPHY

Vaginal Moisturizers

Products such as Replens, Me Again, Vagisil, Feminease, and K-Y SILK-E are designed for vaginal insertion on a regular basis, two or three times a week. They can help keep your partner's vagina moist, but she will probably want to also use a lubricant when you have sex.[28,29]

Vaginal Lubricants

Products such as Slippery Stuff, Astroglide, K-Y Jelly, ID Millennium, Pjur Eros, Pink, and Elegance should be used liberally while you are having sex. Elegance is oil based so it must not be used with condoms.

---

[28] Bachmann and Santen, "Treatment of Vaginal Atrophy" (Apr 4, 2014, UpToDate, www.uptodate.com)

[29] Sobel, "Causes of Vaginitis" (*New England Journal of Medicine*, Vol 337, 1997, p. 1896)

High alert!

With lubricants, it will be much easier for you to get your penis into your partner's vagina. But remember, an estrogen-deficient vagina is less elastic. So you may be excessively stretching your partner's vagina as you take advantage of the easier access. This could be very painful. Don't force it—even if you can—or she's not going to want to do that again! Stop immediately if your partner says that your penis is hurting her. Get off her, and get her and you off in some other way.

Watch for signs of tenderness like your partner grimacing or tensing up when you thrust. I have had women tell me that they are reluctant to disappoint their partner by telling him that it hurts.

Persisting with intercourse when your partner's vagina is tender can cause spasms of the muscles at the vaginal opening, and these spasms can make the tenderness worse and persist even longer. Women avoid sex when they know it's likely to be painful.

Regular Sex

This may also be helpful—yes, I said regular sex.

Women who have sexual intercourse at least once a week have been shown to be less likely to have symptoms of vaginal dryness or tenderness with sex. The improvement in these symptoms is thought to result from the *gentle* stretching of the vagina and the increased blood flow to the vagina that comes with regular sexual intercourse.[30,31] *Please read the above "High alert!" box again!*

Dilators

If your partner is menopausal and has not had sex for several months or longer, her vagina, as a result of the atrophy, may have become too narrow for even gentle, well-lubricated sex.

---

[30] Ibid.

[31] Leiblum, Bachmann, Kemmann, Colburn, and Swartzman, "Vaginal Atrophy in the Postmenopausal Woman. The Importance of Sexual Activity and Hormones" (*Journal of the American Medical Association*, Vol. 249, No.16, 1983, p. 2195)

The best treatment of menopausal vaginal narrowing is vaginal estrogen. But if your partner can't or doesn't want to use estrogen, dilators may help.

Your partner's doctor can provide her with a set of graduated dilators, which look like candles without wicks. Using lots of lubricant, your partner will start with the smaller dilator and gently dilate herself once a day. She will gradually increase the size of the dilator over the next several weeks until she is ready for the real thing—you![32]

WHAT'S NEXT?

Bladder problems in menopause can be quite distressing for women, and these bladder problems can make sex uncomfortable.

This distress and discomfort can affect your partner's well-being, her mood, and her availability for sex. But the good news is that menopausal bladder problems can usually be improved or eliminated. We will discuss this topic in Chapter 7.

---

[32] Carter, Goldfrank, and Schover, "Simple Strategies for Vaginal Health Promotion in Cancer Survivors" (*The Journal of Sexual Medicine*, Vol. 8, No. 2, 2011, p. 549)

Bladder Problems: Put a Little Towel Down

JULIETTE'S STORY

Juliette comes to see me for hot flashes and irregular bleeding. After I do an exam, I discuss the various remedies for hot flashes (detailed in the appendices) with her and schedule her for a test to determine whether her irregular bleeding is of any concern.

Juliette stops me as I'm wrapping up. "Um, Doctor, I have another concern. My husband, Bill, isn't happy with our sex life. I don't know what to do."

I sit back down and ask her to tell me more. "I have to pee more frequently than I used to," she says. "I've been avoiding sex because I often get the strong urge to pee when Bill is thrusting with his, you know, his penis. I'm afraid that he's going to make me pee while we're having sex."

BLADDER PROBLEMS IN MENOPAUSE

Let's take a look at why menopausal women like Juliette may have bladder problems, then we'll get back to Juliette's story.

The urethra (the tube that carries urine from the bladder to the outside) and the bladder floor both sit just in front of the front wall of the vagina. Like the vagina, the urethra and bladder require normal estrogen levels to function properly.

Low estrogen levels can cause thinning, loss of elasticity, loss of muscle tone, and irritability of the tissues of a woman's bladder and urethra and of the muscles and connective tissues that hold the bladder in proper position.

The three most common menopausal bladder problems are stress incontinence, urgency incontinence, and urinary frequency.

Stress Incontinence

If a woman loses urine when she puts stress on her bladder, that's stress incontinence. Women with stress incontinence pee when they cough, sneeze, laugh, lift, squat, run, or jump.

The job of the pelvic floor muscles and connective tissues is to hold the bladder in its normal position when these stresses occur. When the bladder is in normal position, pressures such as those generated by coughing, sneezing, and laughing are transmitted to the bladder outlet and actually help prevent leakage of urine.

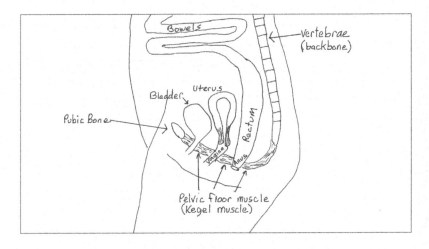

During childbirth, the muscles and connective tissues of the pelvic floor get stretched. These stretched tissues don't always go back to normal after childbirth. But for many women who have given birth, the bladder control problems that result from stretched pelvic floor tissues don't start until they enter menopause. When these women were younger, the pelvic floor muscles and connective tissues were able to hold the bladder in place even though they were damaged during childbirth.

As estrogen levels fall in menopause, these supporting tissues get thin, lose muscle tone, and lose elasticity. They stretch even further, and finally they can no longer hold the bladder in its normal position. Without pelvic floor support, a woman's bladder can sag down so low that pressure from coughing or other stressors can actually push out urine. She may lose urine when she coughs, sneezes, laughs, or lifts.

MAN QUESTION
What can be done to help stress incontinence?
DR. D'S ANSWER
We will talk in detail about vaginal estrogen and Kegel exercises later in this chapter. These two remedies usually help a lot. Some women, though, have such severe stretching of the pelvic floor muscles and connective tissues that they need surgery. We'll talk about that too.

Urgency Incontinence

If a woman gets sudden urges to urinate and the urges are so strong that she can't hold her urine and she pees before she makes it to the bathroom, that's urgency incontinence.

The low levels of estrogen that are in a woman's body during menopause can cause bladder problems similar to those that occur in a woman's vagina in menopause. These changes include thinning, loss of muscle tone, irritability, and loss of elasticity of a woman's bladder wall at its base. When incoming urine stretches a woman's irritable, less pliable bladder, it contracts instead of relaxes as it should. If these involuntary bladder contractions are too strong, the bladder will lose urine.

Urgency incontinence has been called doorknob incontinence. Some menopausal women, when they get home and reach for the front doorknob, will unconsciously send a message to their bladder from their bladder control center in their brain. The message that they unintentionally send to their bladder is that they are almost to the bathroom.

But since they have a thinner, less elastic, more irritable bladder wall, their bladder contracts too soon and they don't make it from the front door to the bathroom.

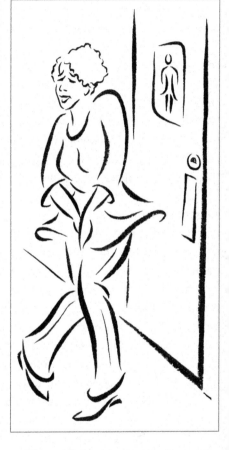

MAN QUESTION
Why do people dance around when they need to urinate?
DR. D'S ANSWER
We learn to dance around to suppress the bladder-emptying reflex when the need to pee is urgent. Moving triggers a reflex that tightens the pelvic floor muscles, which play a major role in bladder control.

Urinary Frequency
WebMD (www.webmd.com) defines urinary frequency as having to urinate more than eight times a day.

There are several different conditions that are associated with frequency, including diabetes, pregnancy, and bladder infections

But in menopause, low estrogen levels cause thinning, loss of muscle tone, irritability, and loss of elasticity at the base of a woman's bladder wall. These changes can result in urinary frequency. It's hard for a woman to get much done when she has to keep running to the bathroom.

DEALING WITH BLADDER PROBLEMS

Fortunately, several approaches are available to improve stress incontinence, urgency incontinence, and urinary frequency.[33]

Vaginal estrogen and *Kegel exercises* can be helpful with all three types of menopausal bladder problems.

Medications can be effective with urgency and frequency but not so much for stress incontinence.

Finally, *surgery* is often the only remedy for stress incontinence. On the other hand, surgery can make urgency or frequency worse.

Vaginal Estrogen

Vaginal estrogen can improve stress incontinence, urgency incontinence, and urinary frequency. Vaginal estrogen is absorbed through the vaginal wall and into the urethra, bladder, and pelvic floor tissues. Estrogen works by restoring the thickness, elasticity, and muscle tone of the bladder base and the pelvic floor muscles and connective tissues. And estrogen lessens bladder wall irritability.

Vaginal estrogen must be prescribed by a doctor, and is not a quick fix by any means. Its effect is subtle, and it takes several weeks to see a noticeable difference.

As discussed in Chapter 6, estrogen can be placed into the vagina in the form of creams, tablets, or a Silastic ring. Vaginal estrogen is not helpful unless it is used regularly, two or three times a week, and on an ongoing basis, pretty much forevermore.

Kegel Exercises

For women who are reading this section, here are some notes that should help with learning and performing Kegel exercises. By using Kegel exercises, women can strengthen the pelvic floor muscles and enhance the communication between the brain and bladder. Often the result is improved bladder control and there are even sexual benefits.

---

[33] Lukacz, "Treatment of Urinary Incontinence in Women" (May 13, 2015, UpToDate, www.uptodate.com)

Most women can make the brain body connection needed to get these muscles to contract; some can't. Technique is everything. To do Kegel exercises correctly, a woman must contract (squeeze) only the pelvic floor muscles—not the abdomen, hip, or thigh muscles.

Three tubes go through the pelvic floor hammock of muscles: the urethra, the vagina, and the rectum (see the drawing on page 44). Squeezing any or all of these openings will produce the same result.

Note 1: Learning Kegels

Here is an excellent technique to use for self-teaching Kegels. Put two fingers into the vagina, and then squeeze around the fingers. If needed, gently jiggle the fingers to help the brain identify which muscles to squeeze.

With the other hand, feel the abdominal, butt, and thigh muscles to be sure that they aren't also tightening. Tightening of these neighboring muscles is called recruiting. Recruiting would make the Kegel squeezes less effective.

After learning to do the Kegel exercises properly, they can be done just about anytime, anywhere. I recommend three sets of ten slow squeezes and three sets of ten rapid squeezes each day, that's sixty squeezes a day. With each slow squeeze, hold to the count of eight. And with each rapid squeeze, squeeze and release immediately.

So, men, if you're at a restaurant and your partner has a look of concentration on her face, she may be doing her Kegel squeezes.

The benefits from Kegels include improvement of stress and urgency incontinence, and urinary frequency. And, oh yes, they can help to make sex more pleasurable.

MAN QUESTION
Huh? Did you say sex?
DR. D'S ANSWER
Yes, Kegel exercises can make sex better for both of you. Your partner can squeeze her vagina around your penis during sex to make it more pleasurable for you. And women tell me that the more they exercise and strengthen their pelvic floor muscles the more they enjoy sex. The Kegel

squeezes enhance a woman's brain body connection to her pelvis. This gives her more pelvic awareness, more sexual pleasure, and more and better orgasms.

Note 2: Kegels for stress incontinence

The stresses of coughing, sneezing, laughing, lifting, squatting, and running can cause urine loss in menopausal women. Women can learn to do an anticipatory Kegel squeeze each time just before coughing, sneezing, or increasing abdominal pressure for any other reason.

The stronger the pelvic floor muscles are, the better the bladder control will be. The better a woman gets at anticipatory squeezes, the less likely she is to leak urine with stress.

Note 3: Kegels for urgency and frequency

Kegel squeezes signal the bladder control center at the bladder outlet to suppress the void reflex and decrease the urge to pee.

The bladder outlet is located where the urethra exits the bladder floor and goes through the pelvic floor muscles. The bladder outlet houses the bladder control center. Women can strengthen the brain body connection to the bladder outlet by doing Kegel squeezes. This will give more conscious control so that the void reflex will be less automatic.

A woman can take advantage of this mechanism by repeatedly doing Kegel squeezes whenever she feels the sensation of wanting to pee. The earlier she begins the squeezes the better control she will have. The stronger her pelvic floor muscles get and the more regularly she uses her Kegel squeezes to suppress the void reflex, the better will be her bladder control.

Medication

Medication is usually not helpful for stress incontinence. But for urinary urgency and frequency, prescription medications such as oxybutynin from the antimuscarinics drug class can make a big difference. These drugs act by relaxing the bladder wall. Common side effects include dry mouth, blurred vision, and constipation. Dose adjustment or changing to a different drug in the antimuscarinic class can help with side effects.

Surgery

Surgery is not recommended for urgency incontinence or frequency and could even make it worse. However, surgery is often the only remedy that will provide satisfactory improvement for stress incontinence.

Stress incontinence results from relaxation and stretching of the muscles and connective tissues that hold a woman's bladder in its normal position. With lengthening of these tissues the bladder slips into a position that is so low that urine is lost during coughing, sneezing, laughing, etc.

During the surgical procedure, a sling usually made of synthetic mesh is placed around the bladder outlet and attached either to the pubic bone or abdominal connective tissue. This corrects the incorrect position of the bladder. Cure rates with surgery for stress incontinence are usually in the 70 to 80 percent range.

MAN QUESTION

So can we get back to how this can improve our sex life?

DR. D'S ANSWER

Let's see what happened with Juliette.

JULIETTE'S STORY—CONTINUED

After talking with Juliette about her being afraid that she would pee during sex with Bill, I prescribe vaginal estrogen. "I recommend that you put estrogen cream into your vagina three nights a week. Replenishing the missing estrogen can improve your bladder symptoms. And estrogen will make your vagina more moist, more elastic, and less likely to be tender during sex."

The lines of tension in Juliette's face relax as she realizes that there is a lot that she can do to improve this awkward situation. "I also recommend that you learn to do Kegel exercises." I give her information on the technique.

"You may feel uncomfortable putting your fingers into your vagina while you're learning to do an effective squeeze." I say. "But this is the best way to learn to do the Kegel exercises effectively."

"I also recommend that you take oxybutynin extended-release tablets by mouth once a day. This will calm your bladder so that your urge to pee is not so strong and you are less likely to lose urine."

"Share your fears with your husband," I say. "I'm guessing that he's feeling unloved and confused right now. When he understands why you've been avoiding sex, he'll be relieved. And I predict that it won't bother him one bit if you leak a little urine during sex. Put a little towel down and enjoy each other."

Juliette returns for follow-up a few weeks later. She's smiling and the tension in her face is gone. "Bill and I are doing a lot better," she says. "I talked with him about how my bladder problems were making me want to avoid sex. Bill told me that he couldn't care less if I leaked some urine during sex." And my bladder is working better since I started the medications and exercises that you recommended."

As I get up to leave, Juliette smiles an embarrassed smile and says, "Bill loves it when I squeeze my vagina around his penis."

WHAT'S NEXT?

A common symptom during menopause is moodiness. Like sex drive, this is a multifaceted problem. Falling hormone levels certainly play a role. But there are many other factors that come in to play.

Take my hand—in a manly way—and let us stroll down this thorny path in Chapter 8. You can make a big difference here. Understanding what your partner is going through will deepen your relationship and lead to better sex.

The Moody Seven

The seven most common situations that I have learned make women moody during menopause are falling hormone levels, physical changes, the empty nest, boomerang kids, lost dreams, decline of intimacy, and fear of aging. In this chapter I'll describe the Moody Seven and offer ideas about what you can do to help.

MAN QUESTION

Ok, this is good. My partner has been really grouchy the past few months, and we don't seem to be as close as we used to be. She has hot flashes once in a while, so I'm thinking she's starting into the change. Our sex life isn't so good either. What can I do to get back my sweetie and our love life?

DR. D'S ANSWER

Good question. In a word, lots. Let's see if we can understand this moodiness thing better. Let's talk about what you can do to help. And let's talk about getting back the sexual intimacy.

Moodiness is commonly seen in menopausal women. The University of Pittsburgh did a moodiness survey of 16,000 women ages forty to fifty-five.[34] About 29 percent of these women complained of feeling tense, depressed, or irritable. They described moodiness to be the most bothersome in the years of early perimenopause (the two to five years before a woman's periods completely stop).

---

[34] Bromberger, Meyer, Kravitz, Sommer, Cordel, Powell, Ganz, and Sutton-Tyrrell, "Psychologic Distress and Natural Menopause: A Multiethnic Community Study" (*American Journal of Public Health*, Vol 91, No. 9, 2001, p. 1435)

MAN QUESTION

I've got my own midlife problems. How can I help my partner with her moodiness? Right now, I either get out of the way or get mad.

DR. D's ANSWER

Well, many of my patients tell me that their man is using the keep-your-distance-or-get-mad approach but with little success.

The likely source of your partner's moodiness is not that simple. That's why I'm going to reveal the seven recurring themes that I have learned make women moody and what might work better than getting out of the way or getting mad.

Read on, oh seeker of the truth.

1. FALLING HORMONE LEVELS

The Issue

Estrogen levels begin a slow, subtle decline in most women when they reach their late thirties. At this age there are seldom any associated symptoms other than, for some women, slight decreases in sex drive and decreased fertility (less likely to get pregnant).

But as a woman gets past age forty, her estrogen levels will fall more and more rapidly. Most women will have very low estrogen levels by age fifty. Certainly your partner's decreasing estrogen levels in menopause can contribute to her moodiness.

A study done in 2001 involving fifty menopausal women with depression showed that 68 percent improved with estrogen therapy. But only 20 percent of the depressed women improved when treated with a placebo (fake estrogen).[35,36]

---

[35] Soares, Almeida, Joffe, and Cohen, "Efficacy of Estradiol for the Treatment of Depressive Disorders in Perimenopausal Women: A Double-Blind, Randomized, Placebo-Controlled Trial" (*Archives of General Psychiatry*, Vol 58, No. 6, 2001, p. 529)

[36] Martin and Barbieri, "Treatment of Menopausal Symptoms with Hormone Therapy" (Jul 7, 2015, UpToDate www.uptodate.com)

The Solution

Your partner may enjoy an improved mood if she chooses to take hormones. Estrogen can be taken by mouth, by skin patch, by skin cream, or it can be put into the vagina.

Estrogen is, hands down, the most effective way to eliminate or at least reduce just about every menopausal symptom, including moodiness.

But studies have shown that women who take hormones in doses high enough to improve general symptoms such as moodiness or hot flashes expose themselves to risks of complications. Current research indicates that the risks of using hormones in menopause are lowest when taken prior to age sixty, when the dose is low, and when they are taken for five years or less. I'll be telling you a lot more about hormones and their associated risks in Appendix 1.

Be a sounding board for your partner as she decides about hormones. But remember, it needs to be her decision. If she decides to take estrogen, you are likely to see an improvement in her disposition. If she decides against estrogen, she may want to consider hormone-free medications, which I describe in Appendix 2, or she may want to try natural remedies, which I discuss in Appendix 3.

2. Physical Changes

"I don't feel pretty. And frankly, Honey, I think you're letting yourself go."

The Issue

Many women in menopause are distressed by the physical changes that they see in the mirror. And they are often disappointed by the changes that they see in their partner.

Women often tell me that they feel less interesting, less beautiful, less desirable, less sexy, and that they feel like they are getting old. They complain that they're getting wrinkles on their face and neck and they're getting droopy breasts. They fight and too often lose the battle against tummy bulge. They spend lots of money at the salon to hide grey, thinning hair.

Too often they catch their partner glancing (or staring) at younger women. They wince when their partner makes insensitive comments like: "You're just getting old, Hon." Or, "Let's face it, you're getting a little chubby." Or, worse yet, "That young babe over there is a real head turner!" Women often tell me that the loss of that pretty-girl look makes them grumpy.

DR. D'S OWN CASE STUDY

I'm not just a gynecologist. I am a husband too. And my wife's experience is a good example of what many women go through. I think that my wife is dazzlingly beautiful and very sexy. I would catch myself staring at her. But I was hiding the stares because I didn't want her to think that I was treating her like a sex object.

She recently shared with me that she often doesn't recognize herself in the mirror. She doesn't like what's happening to her. Her face and her figure don't look like they did when she was in her twenties and thirties. She feels more invisible these days without the admiring glances that she used to get.

I protested and argued that she shouldn't expect to look like she did when she was in her twenties. And doesn't she know how beautiful she is to me? I dropped the ball twice there: not only did I withhold my admiring looks and flirty comments, but when she shared with me how she was feeling, I argued with her instead of telling her that I understood and appreciated what she was going through.

MAN QUESTION

What can I do to help with my partner's self image?

DR. D'S ANSWER

We men often assume that our partner knows how beautiful and desirable she is to us, and so we might not tell her. *Tell her!*

The Solution

Tell your partner how sexy she is! Women tell me that they want to know that they are desirable. So I focus on calling my wife "Beautiful." I greet her with, "Hi, Sexy." I make comments like, "How did I get so lucky that I found you?" *And I mean every word!*

Next, if things aren't going your way, don't pout.

I have had to learn to not get pouty and pull away when my wife is not interested in sexual intimacy. I would protect my feelings in this way. The problem was that by pulling away I was squelching any communications to her that she was desirable to me.

They say that one teaches best that which he needs to learn. I have had to learn to not take my wife's "Not now, honey" as meaning anything other than just that. I have been learning that I need to do my part to keep the relationship good and to find times for intimacy that work for both of us.

And here's another big deal. Some women gain weight during menopause.

If your partner has put on some pounds, she will be painfully aware of it. You don't need to tell her that she needs to go on a diet, and you don't need to make a comment when she's eating ice cream. She's looking for support and affection, not criticism.

Times have changed—or have they? Many years ago my dad used to call my mom Old Sow. He must have thought that he could shame her into losing the weight that had sneaked onto her once-slim body. Mom was usually submissive to my dad, but when she had finally had enough, she got very angry and told him off in no uncertain terms. She made it clear to him that she would no longer tolerate this kind of treatment from him. He didn't ever call her Old Sow again. I'm thinking that my mom didn't feel very sexy when dad talked to her like that.

And even now I have a good friend who sometimes calls his wife Fatty. That can't be good for his sex life either.

So don't call your partner Fatty, like my friend does, or Old Sow, like my dad did.

And take a look at how you support your partner's desire to take off some of that excess weight. So many women have told me that they want to take off weight but their husband or partner won't get on board. He still wants the fatty foods and sweets.

JAN'S STORY

Jan, who lives with her husband Andy, comes for a routine exam.

One of her concerns is weight gain.

"My physique is very important to me," Jan laments. "But Andy insists on having big bags of discount store sweets all over our house. I too often catch myself snacking from them. And Andy won't eat when I prepare healthy, low-sugar foods."

Andy who has a big appetite and a big belly wants Jan to keep her sexy figure but he sabotages her efforts.

Some men subconsciously sabotage their partner's efforts to stay sexy because they don't want other men to be attracted to her. I wonder if that's what Andy is doing.

And Andy's overeating also makes it difficult for Jan to respond to his sexual overtures.

Jan complains, "Andy has gotten so fat that his belly fat hangs down over his lower belly like an apron. His body smells, and since he's been eating sweets all the time his breath smells bad, too. Instead of getting turned on when Andy comes close, I get queasy. And when Andy gets on top of me, he's so heavy that I can't breathe!"

"Jan, you need to have a serious talk with Andy", I say. "Start by telling Andy how much you love him and that you want to reignite the intimacy that you once had."

I go on, "I know this will be very difficult, but you need to tell Andy what you told me about having sweets in the house, about his breath and body odor, and about how his weight smothers you when he's on top trying to make love with you. Can the two of you get on a permanent nutrition and exercise program together?" I discuss options like Weight Watchers and increased physical activity.

It's really difficult to change nutritional and physical activity patterns. But they have a big impact on our health and well being. And our health and physical condition are likely to have an influence on sexual intimacy.

Now that we are in our forties, fifties, sixties, or beyond, let's hope that we have learned to bask in the warm light of love and devotion, which is sweet and sexy in its own way.

So keep the love alive! Don't you want the sweetness and tenderness and romance back? Be sweet and tender and romantic with your partner. Cherish her. See her beauty, regardless of her physical appearance. Tell her repeatedly how beautiful and sexy she is.

And be willing to do what it takes for you to be attractive to her.

3. THE EMPTY NEST

The Issue

Some women tell me that they miss being a mom to their kids. They grieve that their kids are now grown up and gone or going soon.

MAN QUESTION

There's nothing I can do about the empty nest, right?

DR. D'S ANSWER

Not entirely true. Your partner may not even be aware that, on some level, she misses having the kids at home. Be sensitive to that possibility. You may want to ask her if she wishes that she could have another baby. Talking about it can help a lot.

The Solution

Having your kids grow up and move out of the house is a huge change. It helps to talk about it and to make plans to turn this change into a positive one.

Many women get their kid fix by babysitting for their grandkids or volunteering for child care or even getting a puppy. Puppies are cute, and they quickly become part of the family. (And you can board them if you want to travel!)

With the kids out of the house there will likely be lots more discretionary time available. You and your partner may want to start doing activities that until now you didn't have time for. How about boating, hiking, skiing, dancing, or learning to play an instrument?

And how about getting back to regular sexual intimacy by planning sex dates at least once a week. You can make all the noise you want.

4. BOOMERANG BABIES
"They're baaack!"[37]

The Issue

Your partner may be disappointed at how your kids' lives are turning out. She may be stressed and moody because the kids who are now adults have moved back home or need financial assistance way longer than expected.

MAN QUESTION

My partner is not the only one frustrated here. Can I get a crowbar and pry our adult kid out of the house?

---

[37] Michael Grais and Mark Victor, Carol Ann's line from script of *Poltergeist II: The Other Side*, directed by Brian Gibson, produced by Michael Grais and Mark Victor (1986, Beverly Hills, CA, Metro-Goldwyn-Mayer), Film.

Frustrating, huh? Join the club. I've been there too. Below you'll find some thoughts based on personal experience and based on what women have told me over the years.

The Solution

When one (or more) of your kids seems to be stuck in the nest, you might want to notice that they aren't a kid anymore. It helps to remember that you now have an adult family member as a guest in your home.

Can you build a new relationship with your adult kid? Hopefully your relationship with your adult son or daughter will have evolved to the point where you can negotiate new expectations. These new agreements should help to make their stay more tolerable.

My wife and I have two adult daughters. Neither one got stuck in our nest. But they both have boomeranged back at various times. We have had to negotiate new expectations with them. It was hard not to enable their dependence and it was often difficult to communicate what our expectations were.

So team up with your partner. You both may be more moody when an adult offspring is stuck in your nest. This can be a difficult state of affairs. Your approach to this situation may be different from your partner's. Certainly my wife and I have had our disagreements on this subject. Your adult child can easily drive an unintended wedge between you and your partner. I have seen couples at each other's throats over how to handle this situation. Don't let this happen.

My patients have told me that they are way less moody when they are able to team up with their partner to deal with the prolonged dependency of an adult kid. Be each other's support. Talk with your partner about how you, as a couple, want to handle this. Be willing to negotiate and compromise when your opinions differ. Consider professional help if you seem to be stuck.

And the three of you need to have adult conversations to establish a new understanding about how to make it work to have your adult child living with you. Your adult child deserves your respect. But remember, *it's your house!*

MAN QUESTION

Umm, thanks for your sage advice, but its kind of hard to have any privacy when there's an adult kid on the other side of the wall. It was easier to know when we would be alone when the kids were kids. We had control of their schedule then. So what about—you know—sex?

DR. D'S ANSWER

Sex needs to be part of the discussion. Sexual intimacy is a vital ingredient to a healthy relationship for most couples. Having another adult in the home can get in the way. Spontaneous lovemaking is not likely to happen. So plan intimate time with your partner. Find times when the two of you can be alone with no risk of being interrupted.

5. LOST DREAMS

The Issue

Many women age forty and beyond tell me that they are less interested in playing a passive, submissive, or nurturing role in the family. They now need to have their life be a little more about them instead of only about their family. Often they ruminate on missed opportunities in their own career.

A woman once told me, "I didn't expect things to turn out this way. I wanted to be an architect. But I put that dream aside to raise my kids and manage our home. Now I wonder if it's too late."

Stevie Nicks put it this way:

Can I sail through the changing ocean tides?
Can I handle the seasons of my life?
Well, I've been afraid of changing,
'Cause I've built my life around you.
But time makes you bolder.
Even children get older,
And I'm getting older, too. [38]

A frequent question, from women as well as men, is whether hormonal changes have anything to do with the way menopausal women think.

Research shows evidence that there are indeed some changes to women's thought processes in menopause. Estrogen, the nesting hormone, is the dominant hormone in a woman's body in her twenties and thirties, and is thought to enhance a woman's instincts for bearing and raising children. And estrogen is thought to influence women to be more passive and nurturing.

Helen Fisher, a biological anthropologist at Rutgers University, describes estrogen as enabling women to see the big picture, to have strong people skills and verbal skills, and to be imaginative, intuitive, and compassionate.[39]

But when a woman reaches her forties, the estrogen levels in her body begin to decline.

Christiane Northrup, an obstetrician-gynecologist, calls the decreasing dominance of estrogen the "lifting of the hormonal veil."[40] She observes that it's not unusual for a menopausal woman to become

---

[38] Stevie Nicks. "Landslide" on *Fleetwood Mac*. Produced by Fleetwood Mac and Keith Olsen. Reprise Records. 1975.

[39] Helen Fisher, PhD, "What's in a Political Brain?" (*Newsweek*, Nov 5, 2012)

[40] Christiane Northrup, *The Wisdom of Menopause* (New York: A Bantam Book, 2001)

more interested in her own needs, such as career development and realizing dreams and aspirations that are as yet unmet.

Both men and women have in their bodies testosterone, the male hormone, and estrogen, the female hormone. But women have way more estrogen and men have way more testosterone. So when estrogen diminishes in menopausal women, the testosterone, which was always there, becomes more dominant. Helen Fisher describes testosterone qualities as being analytical, tough minded, direct (or even blunt), exacting, skeptical, and competitive. This tipping of the estrogen/testosterone balance influences many women to want to be more worldly and less domestic.[41]

The Solution

Your partner may have dreams and aspirations that she may now fear she will never fulfill. So be your partner's biggest fan. If she wants to make some changes in her life such as going back to school, getting a new job, refocusing on her career, changing careers, or starting her own business, encourage her. Brainstorm with her on ways to finance these new ventures.

MAN QUESTION

Is anything happening to men's hormones at this time in our lives?

DR. D'S ANSWER

Good question! There's often a bit of a role reversal here. In many couples, the woman, with her increasing testosterone influence, wants to get out into the mainstream hubbub at about the same time that her man, with his falling testosterone levels, wants to slow down. We'll talk more about this in the next chapter, which is focused on what we men are going through.

---

[41] Helen Fisher, PhD, "What's in a Political Brain?" (*Newsweek*, Nov 5, 2012)

6. DECLINING INTIMACY

Isn't it a pity
Now, isn't it a shame
How we break each other's hearts
And cause each other pain

How we take each other's love
Without thinking anymore
Forgetting to give back
Isn't it a pity[42]

The Issue

I often hear women confide that they miss the intimacy that they once had in their relationship. They miss the romance and they feel sad and moody as a result.

KAREN'S STORY

Karen and her husband Dan were both close friends of mine. At age fifty, Karen left Dan to be with an old high school boyfriend. I was dismayed. I asked her what had happened.

She told me that she missed the passion and tenderness that weren't there anymore in her marriage. When she and Dan were first dating, they couldn't get enough of each other. "We would often gaze into each other's eyes," she said. "We would talk for hours about pretty much anything. We were so in love."

"But then somehow we became more like roommates. We would talk about family and household matters but otherwise would not pay much attention to each other."

---

[42] George Harrison. "Isn't It a Pity" on *All Things Must Pass*. Produced by George harrison and Phil Spector. Apple, 1970.

> When I had been in their company, I had noticed that there was a kind of cold tone when they talked with each other. Karen was lonely in her home filled with loved ones.
>
> Is there anyway that this sad breakup could have been avoided? Perhaps if Karen and Dan had realized that a loss of intimacy is common in long-term relationships, they could have worked together on recapturing it. Let's take a closer look at how to keep the love alive.

Why does this loss of love and intimacy happen so often?

Let's look at how a new romance is different from an ignored, shriveling, dying romance. In a new romance two people hold each other as the focus in each other's lives. They make time for each other and express interest in each other. They smile and make eye contact. They speak to each other with an affectionate tone of voice. They are sexually intimate on a regular basis.

But the natural passion of a new romance usually lasts only one or two years. After that, life happens. There is a strong tendency for job, home, finances, and kids to pull the passionate couple apart. The couple too often becomes preoccupied keeping all those plates spinning. They unintentionally ignore each other and they ignore their relationship.

When couples drift apart, their sexual relationship suffers. They have less and less sexual intimacy. I have observed that a fading sexual relationship is both a symptom and a cause for the deterioration of romance in many relationships. The ignored relationship shrivels and the sex fades.

Some women blame their loss of sex drive on falling out of love with their mate, when the actual causes are the natural fading of the new relationship passion, the challenges of everyday life, and the natural decline in libido that occurs with falling hormone levels in women in their thirties and beyond.

And the man often pulls away to protect his ego or pride. He has been denied too many times when approaching his partner. Or he has uncertainty about his erections and is keeping his distance to avoid intimacy. It's safer that way. We'll talk lots about erections in the equipment section of Chapter 9, the chapter that's all about changes in men.

The Solution

After observing what happened with Karen and Dan, and with other couples, I came to realize that what may seem like a platitude is actually a powerful truth: Romance in a relationship is like a plant. If it is cared for, paid attention to, fed and watered, it will thrive and grow and be beautiful. If it is ignored, it will shrivel and likely die.

So take care of the romance!

And there is something magical about regular sexual intimacy. In my experience, couples who are sexually intimate on a regular basis tend to keep alive these new romance behaviors.

MAN QUESTION

Okay, Doc, Karen and Dan's story has a spooky familiar ring to it. I can see that my relationship with my partner has been sliding down that same slippery slope. But I don't really know what to do about it.

DR. D'S ANSWER

It's easier to say than do, but that shriveling plant can be revived (maybe not a good metaphor, but I think you see what I mean). You could have a heart-to-heart talk with your partner. Agree to recommit to the romance.

Can you agree to recreate those romantic behaviors? Pay attention to how you talk to your partner, the words you use, and your tone of voice. Have at least one meal together every day. During that meal, leave off the TV and put away the smart phones. Make eye contact with each other and smile. Take walks together, hold hands at least part of the way.

Tell your partner that you want to keep the romance alive. Tell her that you would like to have sex dates with her at least once a week. Set aside time to make love when you aren't tired or distracted. You don't have to be turned on. It's normal for the passion to fade after a year or two in any relationship. But you can revive the intimacy and vulnerability by recommitting to the romance and by making love at least once a week.

In Chapter 10 we'll take a much closer look at what often happens to the sex in a relationship and how to get it back.

7. FEAR OF AGING
"Is this the beginning of the end?"

The Issue
Some women get moody at this time in their lives as they ruminate on their eventual failing health or death. And, we men often have the same ruminations.

Have you noticed that people past age fifty or sixty seem to fall into one of two categories: the defeated and the young at heart.

Those in the first category seem to be defeated by their loss of youth. They often say that they are getting old. They seem to lose interest in life.

But those in the second category manage to take this part of their life as another chapter just as exciting and satisfying as ever before. In fact those in the second group often see this part of their lives as the best ever. This is the time to try new things. And it's the time to give up burdens and worries that are no longer relevant or necessary.

The Solution
I encourage couples at this time in their lives to live each day to the fullest but to shy away from the idea that "our days are numbered." I see that concept as a trap, because it conveys a sense of urgency that saps our aliveness and spontaneity. There is more joy and satisfaction in focusing on each moment for its merits, than in worrying about the future.

The bottom line on the Moody Seven

The falling hormones, the lost youth, the end of parenting as she once knew it, time running out on dreams and aspirations, atrophied romance, the fear of aging—these are the recurring themes that I have come to anticipate when I talk with a woman about being moody at this time in her life.

We men can make a difference when we understand what our partners are going through. A man's responses to these changes will affect his relationship and his sex life. So talk with your partner regularly about what you can do to support her good mood. Be compassionate, and be willing to make some changes in the way you treat each other.

WHAT'S NEXT?

Chapter 9 is about what we men are going through at this time in our lives.

We'll talk about what is happening to our manly hormones. And we'll talk about a very common situation in men forty and beyond, problems getting and maintaining erections. And finally, we'll look at how we as men can decide: Will we live this part of our lives with a young attitude? Or will we stop caring and start the downhill slide?

What About Me, the Man?

"This is a man's, man's, man's world.
But it wouldn't be nothing, nothing without a woman or a girl." [43]

This book focuses on women's issues and how we men can be supportive. But we men have our own issues, which can have a profound impact on our quality of life and our relationship with our partner. So this chapter is all about men.

In the next few pages I'm going to describe how a man's testosterone levels decline as he gets older. I'll explain how these falling testosterone levels can affect a man, and I'm going to discuss the pros and cons of testosterone replacement.

Next we'll take a detailed look at an issue that becomes more likely the older we get, problems getting and keeping an erection. This subject may be a little uncomfortable to read. But I would encourage you to do so. The take-home messages are that there are lots of effective measures that can be taken and that lovemaking need not (dare I say, "should not"?) stop.

And finally we'll discuss the huge impact that we each can have on what our life will be like as we get older. And, yes, this has a lot to do with what our love life will be like.

TESTOSTERONE

Testosterone is the predominant male sex hormone. It influences puberty (sexual maturation), muscle mass and strength, bone strength, general vitality, and sex drive and erections.

---

[43] James Brown and Betty Jean Newsome. *It's a Man's Man's Man's World.* Produced by James Brown. King, 1966.

Andropause (low testosterone) can produce a variety of symptoms. But most of these symptoms can also be explained simply as a result of increasing age.

- Energy levels may decline.
- There may be a decreased desire for sex.
- Men are more likely to have problems getting and maintaining an erection.
- Bone density is lowered, creating a higher risk of fractures.
- Muscle mass and muscle strength are reduced, and body fat tends to increase.
- There is an increased likelihood of anemia, limiting the blood's capacity to carry oxygen.
- Depression and memory loss are more likely.
- Men are more prone to obesity, diabetes, high blood pressure, and earlier mortality.

In men past age forty, testosterone levels typically decline at about 1 percent per year.[44, 45]

Effectiveness of Testosterone Replacement

The television ads for "Low T" say that taking testosterone helps with the symptoms mentioned in the list above. But unfortunately the ads are misleading. Many men after age forty have these symptoms regardless of their testosterone levels. And clinical observations don't clearly demonstrate that taking supplemental testosterone helps. [46, 47, 48]

---

[44] Snyder, "Overview of Testosterone Deficiency in Older Men" (Jun 17, 2014, UpToDate, www.uptodate.com)

[45] Wu, Tajar, Pye, Silman, Finn, O'Neill, Bartfai, Casanueva, Forti, Giwercman, Huhtaniemi, Kula, Punab, Boonen, Vanderschueren, and European Male Aging Study Group, "Hypothalamic-Pituitary-Testicular Axis Disruptions in Older Men are Differentially Linked to Age and Modifiable Risk Factors: The European Male Aging Study" (*Journal of Clinical Endocrinology & Metabolism*, Vol 93, No. 7, 2008, p. 2737)

[46] Snyder, "Overview of Testosterone Deficiency in Older Men" (Jun 17, 2014, UpToDate, www.uptodate.com)

What does the evidence tell us about the effectiveness of testosterone replacement?

- Fatigue: There is no good evidence that testosterone replacement improves fatigue.
- Sexual function: Testosterone use may increase libido (sex drive). But there is little or no improvement of erectile function (ability to get and keep an erection) and little or no improvement of sexual satisfaction.[49]
- Bone density: Testosterone shots (high doses) will improve bone density but only in men with very low testosterone. Transdermal testosterone (testosterone that you put on your skin) does not improve bone density.[50]
- Muscles: Testosterone use has been shown to increase muscle mass and decrease fat mass.[51] But testosterone has not been shown to improve muscle strength in men over sixty-five.[52]
- Anemia: Testosterone does improve anemia, but only in men with

---

[47] Liverman and Blazer (Eds), *Testosterone and Aging: Clinical Research Directions.* (Washington, DC: National Academies Press, 2004)

[48] Snyder, "Overview of Testosterone Deficiency in Older Men" (Jun 17, 2014, UpToDate, www.uptodate.com)

[49] Isidori and Lenzi, "Testosterone Replacement Therapy: What We Know Is Not Yet Enough" (*Mayo Clinic Proceedings*, Vol 82, No. 1, 2007, pp. 11–3)

[50] Tracz, Sideras, Boloña, Haddad, Kennedy, Uraga, Caples, Erwin, and Montori, "Testosterone Use in Men and Its Effects on Bone Health. A Systematic Review and Meta-analysis of Randomized Placebo-Controlled Trials" (*Journal of Clinical Endocrinology & Metabolism*, Vol 91, No. 6, 2006, pp. 2011–6)

[51] Bhasin, Cunningham, Hayes, Matsumoto, Snyder, Swerdloff, and Montori, "Testosterone Therapy in Adult Men with Androgen Deficiency Syndromes: An Endocrine Society Clinical Practice Guideline" (*Journal of Clinical Endocrinology & Metabolism*, Vol. 91, No. 6, 2006, p. 1995)

[52] Snyder, Peachey, Hannoush, Berlin, Loh, Lenrow, Holmes, Dlewati, Santanna, Rosen, and Strom, "Effect of Testosterone Treatment on Body Composition and Muscle Strength in Men Over 65 Years of Age" (*Journal of Clinical Endocrinology & Metabolism*, Vol. 84, No. 8, 1999, p. 2647)

severe testosterone deficiency.[53]

- Depression: Two small studies (the smaller the study, the less reliable the results) suggest that testosterone use may improve depression.[54]

- Memory loss: I could find no studies that demonstrate that using testosterone improves memory.

- Diabetes, high blood pressure, and earlier mortality: Testosterone has not been shown to improve or prevent these medical conditions.

Risks of Testosterone Replacement

We have seen that testosterone supplements may not be effective in treating many of the conditions we observe in men over forty. And unfortunately there are some significant risks in raising testosterone levels through supplementation.

- Benign prostatic hyperplasia (BPH): The prostate gland surrounds a man's urethra[55] just as it comes out of the bladder. A man's prostate will probably enlarge gradually as he gets older. BPH is a condition where the prostate has gotten so large that it narrows the urethra and causes difficulty urinating. BPH is common in men past age forty. Fifty percent of all men will have symptomatic BPH by age sixty, and 80 percent of men will have BPH symptoms by age eighty.[56] Testosterone therapy is suspected of making BPH

---

[53] Snyder, Peachey, Berlin, Hannoush, Haddad, Dlewati, Santanna, Loh, Lenrow, Holmes, Kapoor, Atkinson, and Strom, "Effects of Testosterone Replacement in Hypogonadal Men" (*Journal of Clinical Endocrinology & Metabolism*, Vol. 85, No. 8, 2000, p. 2670)

[54] Shores, Kivlahan, Sadak, Li, and Matsumoto, "A Randomized, Double-Blind, Placebo-Controlled Study of Testosterone Treatment in Hypogonadal Older Men with Subthreshold Depression (Dysthymia or Minor Depression)" (*Journal of Clinical Psychiatry*, Vol. 70, No. 7, 2009, pp. 1009–16)

[55] The urethra is the tube that goes from your bladder to the tip of your penis. It empties the urine out of your bladder.

[56] Berry, Coffey, Walsh, et al., "The Development of Human Benign Prostatic Hyperplasia with Age" (*Journal of Urology*, Vol. 132, 1984, p. 474)

worse, but this has not been proven. Studies are ongoing.

- Prostate cancer: Testosterone therapy is thought to have the potential of increasing the risk of prostate cancer, but this has not been proven. Prostate-specific antigen (PSA) is a protein produced by the prostate. When PSA levels are increased, the risk of prostate cancer is higher. PSA levels are higher in men taking testosterone but only slightly higher.

- Sleep apnea: In this condition, the airway passage from the nose and mouth to the lungs partially or completely collapses during sleep. This results from relaxation of the dilator muscles that ordinarily keep the airway open. Snoring, intermittent breathing, choking, and gasping at night are common symptoms of sleep apnea. Testosterone therapy may increase the likelihood of this condition. Some studies suggest that sleep apnea worsens in men taking testosterone. Other studies don't confirm this.[57]

- Erythrocytosis: This is a condition where the number of red blood cells increases to an abnormally high concentration (the opposite of anemia). Men with erythrocytosis have a higher risk of death from heart attacks. Studies clearly show that about 25 percent of men who take testosterone will develop erythrocytosis.[58]

MAN QUESTION

Doc, after five pages of detailed discussion, are you saying that while low testosterone could be causing me some problems, I probably shouldn't take testosterone?

DR. D'S ANSWER

---

[57] Calof, Singh, Lee, Kenny, Urban, Tenover, and Bhasin, "Adverse Events Associated with Testosterone Replacement in Middle-Aged and Older Men: A Meta-Analysis of Randomized, Placebo-Controlled Trials" (*Journals of Gerontology, Series A: Biological Sciences and Medical Sciences*, Vol. 60, No. 11, 2005, p. 1451)

[58] Hajjar, Kaiser, and Morley, "Outcomes of Long-Term Testosterone Replacement in Older Hypogonadal Males: A Retrospective Analysis" (*Journal of Clinical Endocrinology & Metabolism*, Vol 82, No. 11, 1997, p. 3793)

Uh, kind of. As we men get older, our testosterone levels naturally fall. The declining testosterone levels may produce some symptoms. Unfortunately, unless testosterone levels are severely depressed, replacement does not always improve the symptoms. And testosterone replacement can create its own set of problems.

FOLLOW-UP MAN QUESTION

OKAY! OKAY! SO WHAT DO I DO?! (Sorry to shout but this seems to be pretty important!)

DR. D.'S ANSWER

All of these symptoms can be improved with other measures such as healthy diet, regular gentle exercise, and healthy sleep practices. This is a wake-up call! We men need to pay serious attention to taking care of our health. Medications are not always the best approach. If these measures aren't sufficient, you may want to consult with your doctor.

FOLLOW-UP TO THE FOLLOW-UP MAN QUESTION

OKAY! I'll have smoothies. I'll get an elliptical trainer. I'll get regular sleep. But I still think that I need testosterone! What do I do?

DR. D'S ANSWER

If you have symptoms suggestive of low testosterone (low libido, low energy, depressed mood, osteoporosis, or anemia), ask your doctor to measure your serum total testosterone. If the testosterone levels in your serum are consistently less than 200 mg/dl and no pituitary or testicular abnormalities are found, testosterone therapy may need to be considered. But given the uncertain outcomes, and the possible risks of taking testosterone, you should very carefully review the likely benefits and potential side effects and risks of testosterone replacement with your doctor.

THE EQUIPMENT

PSSST, MAN QUESTION

Uh, here's the thing. My equipment isn't working as well as it used to. Frankly, I've been avoiding sex. Sometimes I think that I unconsciously approach my partner for sex at a time that I know she won't want it. Maybe that allows me to blame her for our lack of passion.

DR. D'S ANSWER

Problems getting and keeping an erection are actually quite common.

- About 40 percent of men in their forties have problems getting or keeping an erection.
- After age forty, the percentage of men with erection problems is about the same as their age. So 50 percent at age fifty, 60 percent at age sixty, and on from there.[59]

PATTY'S STORY

Patty comes to see me for a checkup.

I routinely ask women during checkups whether they are in a sexual relationship. When asked this question, Patty's head drops and her eyes moisten. "My husband and I haven't had sex for over a year." I expect her to cry any second. "He told me that he didn't want to have sex with me any more because I was getting fat. But after I took off the extra pounds, he still hasn't been interested."

"What was the sex like when you did have it?" I ask.

"Well, it was great for me, but there were times when he couldn't get it up. And there were other times when he wouldn't stay hard. I didn't really care so much about that, but it seemed to bother him a lot."

"I wonder if your husband is avoiding sex with you because of his problems getting and keeping an erection," I say. "Do you think that he could

---

[59] Feldman, Goldstein, Hatzichristou, Krane, and McKinlay, "Impotence and Its Medical and Psychosocial Correlates: Results of the Massachusetts Male Aging Study" (*Journal of Urology*, Vol. 151, No. 1, 1994, p. 54)

have made the comments about your weight in order to avoid the embarrassment of his 'poor performance'?"

Patty didn't respond.

"Have a heart-to-heart talk with your husband," is my advice. "Tell him that you love him dearly and that you don't really care if he gets hard or stays hard. Tell him that you miss the sweetness and tenderness that you had when you were sexually intimate. Tell him that you want to have naked time with him. Caressing and loving is what you want, hard-on or not. Tell him that your gynecologist suggested that he see a urologist if he wants help with his erections. There are many remedies that can help."

I hope that Patty takes my advice. And I hope that her husband does too.

Read on to see what the possibilities are.

WHAT WOMEN WANT

In her book *Women's Bodies, Women's Wisdom,*[60] Christiane Northrup points out that less than 25 percent of women reach orgasm with penile–vaginal intercourse. It's a ruse, guys; we men have been fooled into thinking that we need a big erection to please a woman.

Women want intimacy, they want tenderness, they want pleasure, and they want orgasms. But an erect penis is not a requirement. It's a way bigger deal to us men than it is to most women, except for those women who have bought into the same lie. Let's get over ourselves and have fun with each other instead of stressing over how big an erection we can get.

But women often do need reassurance. They need to know that when their man is having a problem with erections, this does not mean that he is no longer attracted to her or that he is having an affair.

---

[60]Christiane Northrup, *Women's Bodies, Women's Wisdom* (New York: A Bantam Book, 2010)

In real life, sexual intimacy looks very different from what we read about in books and what we see in movies or on TV.[61] Whatever way you and your partner choose to express sexual intimacy behind closed doors—erection or not—is just fine as long as you don't compare yourselves unfavorably to the movie-dream-world fantasy.

When a man avoids sex because of performance concerns, the relationship often becomes less sweet, romantic, intimate, and fun. You can do your magic in the sheets with your fingers, your tongue, and sex toys.

MAN QUESTION
Thanks for your soothing words, but when the time is right, I really do want my equipment to work. What can I do?
DR. D'S ANSWER
First let's talk about what an erection is and then I'll give you some ideas that should help.

MAN QUESTION
What happens when a man gets an erection?
DR. D'S ANSWER
When a man gets sexually excited, the arteries that send blood to his penis expand and more blood flows in. At that same time, the veins that drain his penis clamp down so that the blood can't drain out. This makes his penis fill with blood, expand, and get firm. Boom! He has an erection.

MAN QUESTION
Great, thanks for the lesson in hydraulics, but what can be done to make my equipment work better?

---

[61] Rachel Hills, *The Sex Myth: The Gap Between Our Fantasies and Reality* (New York: Simon & Schuster, 2015)

79

DR. D'S ANSWER

There are lots of ways for you to enhance your erections. There are pills, urethral suppositories, shots, constriction rings, vacuum pumps, and surgery. And there are other remedies that don't work so well. Let's take a look at what's available. Keep trying until you find one that works for you.

MEDICAL REMEDIES TO ENHANCE ERECTIONS

Supplementing Testosterone

As we discussed, testosterone patches, pills, and shots have been shown to increase sex drive in men with abnormally low levels of this male hormone. But there is no good evidence that they improve a man's likelihood of getting and keeping an erection.[62]

Erection Pills

Do the pills work? And if so how?

Pill choices include Viagra (sildenafil), Levitra or Staxyn (vardenafil), and Cialis or Adcirca (tadalafil). These erection enhancer pills really do work in 69 to 89 percent of men.[63] With these prescription drugs you are more likely to get hard even if you are nervous: and you'll stay hard longer. Another plus is that most men using these drugs are also less likely to ejaculate prematurely. These pills don't cause an erection unless you are sexually aroused, so don't worry about going around looking like you have a banana in your pants.

---

[62] Tsertsvadze, Fink, Yazdi, MacDonald, Bella, Ansari, Garritty, Soares-Weiser, Daniel, Sampson, Fox, Moher, and Wilt, "Oral Phosphodiesterase-5 Inhibitors and Hormonal Treatments for Erectile Dysfunction: A Systematic Review and Meta-Analysis" (*Annals of Internal Medicine*, Vol. 151, No. 9, 2009, p. 650)

[63] Cunningham, "Treatment of Male Sexual Dysfunction" (Sept 16, 2015, UpToDate, www.uptodate.com)

When and how should these medications be taken?

Viagra and Levitra take effect about thirty minutes after being swallowed with their greatest effect in about one hour. Duration of effect is about four hours.

Cialis has onset of effect in thirty minutes to one hour with peak effect at one to six hours. Its greatest effect is during the first eighteen hours but it continues to have significant effect for a full thirty-six hours.

Studies have shown that a half dose of Cialis can be taken as a daily pill. This may allow you to be ready anytime.[64]

You may want to try Viagra or Levitra first and see how you do with the side effects. Cialis is only half gone after eighteen hours. Also, Levitra and Viagra have a faster onset of action.

What about dosage?

All three come in three dose strengths. With all three the cost per tablet is similar regardless of strength. They are expensive; so ask your doctor to prescribe the middle or highest strength so that you can get a pill cutter and cut them in half for dose adjustment.

Are there any side effects?

Possible side effects of these drugs include headaches, heartburn, nausea, diarrhea, flushing (red face), dizziness, insomnia, fever, blurred or blue vision, and light sensitivity. Less likely side effects, in the 1 to 10 percent range, include skin rash, anemia, liver problems, muscle aches, paresthesia (tingling, itching, or burning of the skin), difficulty breathing, nosebleed, and nasal congestion. As with any drug, there are myriad other potential side effects.

---

[64] Porst, Giuliano, Glina, Ralph, Casabé, Elion-Mboussa, Shen, and Whitaker, "Evaluation of the Efficacy and Safety of Once-a-Day Dosing of Tadalafil 5mg and 10mg in the Treatment of Erectile Dysfunction: Results of a Multicenter, Randomized, Double-Blind, Placebo-Controlled Trial" (*European Urology*, Vol. 50, No. 2, 2006, p. 351)

Priapism is another risk. Priapism is a prolonged erection (greater than four hours). This occurs in less than 2 percent of users. Sounds like a dream come true, right? Wrong! Priapism is usually painful and can cause injury to your penis and can result in permanent difficulties having an erection.

Priapism is a medical emergency but can be treated effectively if there is no delay in getting medical attention. If your erection lasts for more than three hours, head for your doctor's office or the emergency room. It's worth the embarrassment.

In summary: If you want help getting and maintaining erections, Viagra, Levitra, and Cialis can make a huge difference. And if the pills are not for you or don't work for you, your urologist can offer you many other remedies to help the equipment work.

Suppositories and Injections

Urethral suppositories may work when Viagra, Levitra, and Cialis don't work or aren't tolerated. Urethral suppositories are tiny waxy alprostadil pellets that you insert into your urethra just before sex. The erection lasts for about an hour, and the suppositories are effective in about two-thirds of men.[65]

Penile injections are drugs (alprostadil and VIP/phentolamine) that you inject into the body of your penis using a syringe and a tiny needle. I know that this sounds gruesome, but if you are motivated, it will get easier each time you inject yourself. The erection lasts for about an hour and the injections are effective in about 86 percent of men.[66]

Side effects of suppositories and injections include about a 50 percent likelihood of penile or testicular pain. Headache, dizziness,

---

[65] Cunningham, "Treatment of Male Sexual Dysfunction" (Sept 16, 2015, UpToDate, www.uptodate.com)

[66] Linet and Ogrinc, "Efficacy and Safety of Intracavernosal Alprostadil in Men with Erectile Dysfunction. The Alprostadil Study Group" (*New England Journal of Medicine*, Vol. 334, No. 14, 1996, p. 873)

rapid heartbeat, and hypertension are also side effects, though less likely.

Priapism has been reported in 6 to 11 percent of men using the suppositories and injections. Again, an erection lasting more than three to four hours can injure your penis and should be considered a medical emergency.

The Penile Prosthesis

The prosthesis is a device that can be surgically implanted into your penis. There are two types of prostheses.

The semirigid prosthesis is a two-piece set of bendable rods that are surgically implanted, one on each side of your penis. Once the rods are placed you will have a permanent erection. You bend your penis up for sex and bend it back down against your leg the rest of the time.[67]

The inflatable prosthesis is a two-piece set of hollow cylinders that are surgically implanted, one on each side of your penis. Your penis will look close to normal except when you inflate the cylinders with saline (salt water).

A squeeze pump is placed in your scrotum next to one of your testicles. You can achieve an erection by repeatedly squeezing the pump. And—depending on the design—you can deflate it either by bending your penis or pushing a valve mechanism on the pump. There is a 90 percent satisfaction rate with the inflatable prostheses.[68]

NONMEDICAL REMEDIES TO ENHANCE ERECTIONS

Most of the nonprescription remedies that we all see on television, in spam, magazine ads, newspaper ads, and in adult sex shops are a waste of your money. However, there are a few exceptions.

---

[67] Wilson, "Penile Prostheses at the Millennium" (*Contemporary Urology*, Vol 13, 2001, p. 35)

[68] Levine, Estrada, and Morgentaler, "Mechanical Reliability and Safety of, and Patient Satisfaction with the Ambicor Inflatable Penile Prosthesis: Results of a 2 Center Study" (*Urology*, Vol. 166, No. 3, 2001, pp. 932–7)

I am not a fan of counseling for erection difficulties. But the two devices that I will describe do work.

Counseling

Our culture (and most other cultures) unfairly—and cruelly, I think—link a man's erections to his manhood. Consequently, most men get very upset when they don't get an erection when they expect one.

A popular approach to sexual problems has been counseling. In my experience, counseling is usually not helpful for erection problems, and it is time consuming and expensive. There is subtext here that infers that this man will be getting erections just as soon as he starts thinking right. It seems to me that this would be like getting counseling for visual problems when, really, what you need is to get some glasses.

My suggestion is that if you don't get or keep a satisfactory erection during sex, use your tongue, fingers, or a sex toy to please your partner. You can also try the two types of erection aids that we are discussing here.

Constriction Rings

Constriction rings, or cock rings, are stretchable bands that are placed around the base of your penis. They need to be tight enough to block your penis from draining its blood but not so tight that the blood can't flow in to fill it up. The penile artery fills your penis with blood and the elastic band prevents the blood from draining back out. This works because the pressure of the blood in the inflow arteries is quite a bit higher than the pressure in the outflow veins.

While it works just fine for a relatively short period, you should not leave a cock ring in place for more than thirty minutes or so. Prolonged restriction of the blood flow could injure your penis. And it is critically important that the band can be stretched or cut, to be absolutely sure that you can remove it. You may want to do some manscaping. Otherwise hairs can get pulled during placement and removal of the band.

You should be able to ejaculate with the band in place, but your ejaculation fluid may not come out until the ring is removed. A little experimentation will quickly give you an idea of the effectiveness of this method and how to make it work best for you.

Cock rings can be purchased at adult sex shops or online.

Vacuum Erection Device (VED)

A VED is a hollow cylinder that you place over your penis. Vacuum is gradually applied until your penis fills with blood and becomes erect. A constriction ring is then placed at the base of your penis to prevent it from deflating. As I mentioned above, the constriction ring must be stretchable so that it can be removed to allow for your penis to drain itself.

Success with this method has been reported as anywhere from 25 to 83 percent.[69] There is a learning curve here. Practice with it in private until you get it to work for you.

VEDs can also be purchased at sex shops and online. Some medical insurance plans will pay for all or part of their purchase cost if prescribed by a doctor.

THINK AND ACT YOUNG

In an article in the *New York Times,* Bruce Grierson describes studies being conducted by Ellen Langer, professor of psychology at Harvard. These studies suggest that our mind-set can have a dramatic effect on how we age. Study participants who learn to see themselves as young and strong actually test younger. They are more supple and show greater manual dexterity, improved posture, better memory, and improved sight.[70] Everything that you do to enhance your vitality will

---

[69] Tay and Lim, "A Prospective Trial with Vacuum-Assisted Erection Devices" (*Annals of Academy Medicine Singapore*, Vol. 24, No. 5, 1995, p. 705)

[70] Grierson, "What if Age Is Nothing but a Mind-Set?" (*The New York Times*, Oct 22, 2014)

make you feel better and make you more sexually attractive to your mate.

Testosterone, the aggression or dominance hormone, begins to decline in most men at about the same time that a woman's estrogen level is falling. As a result, many men at this age become—as Dr. Northrup puts it—world-weary. They become more interested in staying home at the time that their partners want to get out and try new things.[71]

My friend Jerilyn shared with me that she knows several men who were great companions until they got to middle age. They now have become what she labels "dork chops." They used to have a sunny outlook but now they more often are cranky. They complain that they're getting old and seem less interested in living life to its fullest. They say that they're too tired. They used to look great but now they are paying less attention to their fitness, dress, and hygiene.

But are we doomed to becoming dork chops at this time in our lives? I don't think so!

You can go to extremes with impossible schemes.
You can laugh when your dreams fall apart at the seams.
And life gets more exciting with each passing day.
And love is either in your heart, or on its way

. . . . .
And here is the best part, you have a head start,
If you are among the very young at heart.[72]

Here are some keys to thinking young:
- Stay active, involved, and enthusiastic. Get involved in making a difference. Give back by volunteering.

---

[71] Christiane Northrup, *The Wisdom of Menopause* (New York: A Bantam Book, 2001)
[72] Frank Sinatra, vocal performance of "Young at Heart" by Johnny Richards and Carolyn Leigh. 1953.

- Generate and show enthusiasm about getting out to the theater, or to a restaurant, or being with friends.
- Be active physically. (See my Dick Van Dyke story below.)
- Take care of your health, appearance, and hygiene.
- Learn new things.
- Watch your mood. If you catch yourself being grumpy, at least communicate to your partner how you feel so that she doesn't take your moodiness personally.
- Watch what you think and say about your age. Don't start down that I'm-getting-old path.

And keep moving! Dick Van Dyke recently appeared on Conan on TBS Television. This eighty-nine-years-young dynamo came dancing out onto the stage and looked great. He then proceeded to teach Conan a few dance steps.

Van Dyke shared that his agent had suggested that he write a book about his secret for staying young. He told his agent that the book would need to be only two words long. It would say: "Keep moving!" Now those are words to live by!

"There are times when I really don't feel like getting out of bed," he said. "That's when I remind myself of my decision to keep moving whether I feel like it or not. So I get moving, and I feel better and better as the day goes on!"

NEWSFLASH: I just discovered that Van Dyke has just released a new book, *Keep Moving*.[73]

---

[73] Dick Van Dyke, *Keep Moving and Other Tips and Truths About Aging* (New York, Weinstein Books, 2015)

Sex, Intimacy, and Menopause

WHAT'S NEXT?

The next chapter is all about—wait for it—sex! Women and their partners typically go through sexual changes both individually and in their relationships with each other during the menopausal years.

How these sexual changes affect the two of you is up to you; it's a decision you must make. Will you decide that this is the end of your love life and, as a result, become roommates or go separate ways? Or will you, as a couple, decide to embrace the changes and keep the intimacy alive and well, in its new form.

Actually, I already know what you have decided. You wouldn't be reading this book were you not determined to keep the love alive.

CHAPTER 10

Sex—Let's Keep the Love Alive!

NANCY'S STORY

Nancy, a forty-eight-year-old woman, comes in for a checkup. She speaks softly with muted emotion.

"Doctor, I have no sex drive. My husband and I hardly ever make love. Mark usually comes on to me for sex after we go to bed. By that time I'm too tired. I just want to go to sleep. But regardless of when he wants it, I'm really never in the mood."

I ask Nancy what it's like to have sex with Mark.

"Oh, it's fine. I actually enjoy it once we're doing it. But afterwards I'm back to not really being interested."

"Tell me about your relationship with Mark."

"We get along just fine." She sounds defeated.

"Are the sweetness and tenderness still there?" I ask.

"Well no, not really. We're more like good friends now."

"Do you miss the sweetness and tenderness and romance that you had during the earlier years of your relationship?"

"Yes I do." There is no hesitation to her response.

We'll come back to Nancy and Mark later in the chapter. Does their story ring true to you at all? I often hear this story, or something like it, from women ages forty and beyond. It seems to be more the rule than the exception. But does it have to be like this? I don't think so.

Can your love life make a comeback? *Yes it can!*

Let's talk about five steps that you and your partner can take to keep the love alive, and get intimacy and sex back into your relationship.

1. START WITH GOOD HYGIENE

In forty years of practicing gynecology a common theme that I have heard from women is that their man has let his hygiene lapse.

- He doesn't shower and shave regularly.
- He has hairs growing out of his nose.
- He doesn't keep his teeth clean and white.
- He farts and belches loudly and proudly.
- He wears old, shabby clothes.
- He smokes or chews.
- He has gained a lot of weight.

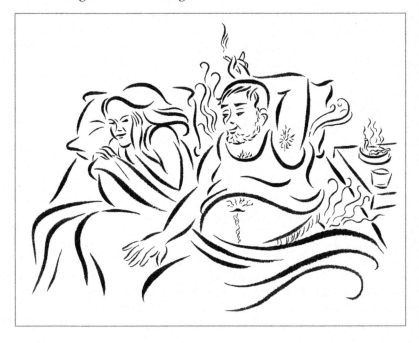

Women tell me that they're more interested in sex when their man's breath and body smell good and when he pays attention to his appearance. C'mon guys, how hard is it to lather up the old toothbrush, or hit the shower after work?

When I catch myself slipping into my "she's-my-roommate" mode, it helps to remind myself that my wife is my Love and my Lover. This motivates me to take care of my teeth and my breath, to shower and shave even on my days off, to keep my body gases to myself, and to be mindful of my appearance.

I'm not saying that we men can't be comfortable when we're at home. I'm just sayin'.

2. FACE UP TO FALLING HORMONES.

Lower sex drive is associated with lower estrogen. Many women experience diminishing sex drive starting as early as in their thirties. And when they hit menopause, their sex drive often drives off a cliff.

This is normal. Part of a woman's libido is hormone dependent. As her estrogen levels fall the hormonal component of her libido is also likely to fall.[74, 75]

The trick is for us men to not get our feelings hurt if our partner seems uninterested. It may have nothing to do with us. When we men get our feelings hurt, we sometimes pout or withdraw.

STEVE'S STORY

My good friend Steve told me that he hadn't touched his wife for several weeks because she wasn't responding to his sexual overtures. I shared with him that her lack of interest in sex could be hormonal and that withdrawing from her was the worst thing he could do.

My advice to Steve was that he tell his wife that he gets his feelings hurt when she's not interested in making love. He could tell her that he's reading a book that explains that her lack of interest could be hormonal and that he'll try to be more understanding and not pull away from her. He could tell her

---

[74] Dennerstein, Dudley, Hopper, and Burger, "Sexuality, Hormones and the Menopausal Transition" (*Maturitas*, Vol. 26, No. 2, 1997, p. 83)

[75] Shifren, "Sexual Dysfunction in Women: Epidemiology, Risk Factors, and Evaluation" (May 20, 2014, UpToDate, www.uptodate.com)

> that he wants to keep their romance alive, that he would like to plan to have a sex date with her once a week, and that he hopes she is open to that.

Falling estrogen levels in menopause can make a woman less likely to be sexually aroused. But being aroused is not a requirement for sexual intimacy. When two people decide that they want to reestablish the romance, intimacy, and tenderness in their relationship, regular sex—aroused or not—can be the catalyst. Read on. We'll talk lots more about this.

3. BE A PARTNER

What is the power dynamic in your relationship? Are you the boss? Estrogen, the primary female hormone, is known to influence a woman to be more passive and nurturing.

But as she enters her menopausal years, her estrogen levels begin to fall and she is less likely to tolerate a relationship with a dominating partner. Many relationships deteriorate at about this time in life if the man persists at being a controller/dominator.

So be a partner, not a dominator. You could be a controller/dominator if:

- You make pretty much all of the decisions.
- You always get the last word.
- You often criticize your partner.
- You criticize her friends and family.
- You get jealous.
- You get ugly when you don't get your way.

So don't be a caveman. Take an honest look at how you relate to your partner. If you are controlling or dominating, that's not sexy. Equal power in a relationship begets vulnerability and intimacy.

But normalizing power dynamics that may have been out of balance for years may not be easy. Some couples find that professional marriage counseling helps at this point. Or consider whether you might benefit from individual counseling.

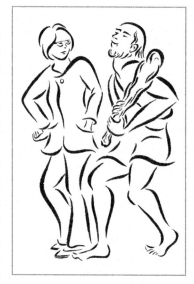

Of course there's another side to the coin: is your mate the boss? As we discussed earlier in this chapter, at about the same time in life when a woman's passive, nurturing estrogen levels begin to fall, a man's aggression/dominance testosterone levels are also falling. Some couples reverse roles. The man may become less dominant and more passive, and the woman may become less passive and more dominant. Ask yourself these questions:

- Does your partner make pretty much all the decisions?
- Do you defer to your partner when it comes to decisions about whom to socialize with?
- Who decides which restaurant to go to? What TV show or movie to watch? When to turn off the TV? When to go to bed?
- Does your partner decide when and where to go on vacation?
- How about what furniture to get? Where to place the furniture? Which way to go when you take walks?

While your partner doesn't want someone who always argues, complains, or resists, nor is she likely to want someone who is entirely compliant and easily overpowered in arguments and decisions. You're looking for a respectful and caring dynamic with equal give and take.

Again, consider getting counseling if you get angry at your partner and at yourself if she dominates in the relationship.

But is the sex really more frequent and better in equal power relationships? In a *New York Times* article,[76] Lori Gottlieb referred to studies that suggest that sex may not be more frequent or more satisfying, but that there were certainly some positive recurring themes in more equal relationships: couples were closer and happier, they were more satisfied with the marriage, and divorce was less likely.

In an established relationship, equal or not, the frequency of sex—especially spontaneous sex—is likely to diminish with time. But if the relationship is egalitarian (has equal power dynamics), resentment is less likely and quality communication is way more likely. Couples who treat each other with mutual appreciation and respect set the stage for increased intimacy.

This is where sex dates come into play. Use your open communication line to plan sex dates at least once a week. This will keep the romance, vulnerability, and intimacy alive. See the "Make Sex Dates" section later in this chapter for more on this very important topic.

Be honest with each other about how you can be better partners, and don't expect your partner to take care of you. Do you make messes and expect your partner to clean them up? Or do you participate—without whining—in routine tasks like cooking, doing the dishes, shopping, laundry, and walking the dog? When you do, you are working as a team. There will likely be less resentment and better communication. Did I mention sex dates?

4. TAKE CARE OF THE ROMANCE

The first one or two years of most relationships are all about the passion of newness. But, especially after the newness wears off, relationships need attention. The romance must be cared for.

---

[76] Gottlieb, "Does a More Equal Marriage Mean Less Sex?" (*The New York Times*, Feb 6, 2014)

It seems to me that: If there's no romance, there's no sex. If there's no sex, there's no romance!

So share activities you both like: eat meals together; take walks together; spend time together without the TV, computer, or smartphones.

Remember "The Piña Colada Song"?

So I waited with high hopes and she walked in the place.
I knew her smile in an instant. I knew the curve of her face.
It was my own lovely lady, and she said, "Oh it's you?"
Then we laughed for a moment and I said, "I never knew
That you like Piña Coladas, getting caught in the rain,
And the feel of the ocean, and the taste of champagne.
If you like making love at midnight in the dunes of the Cape
You're the lady I've looked for, come with me and escape." [77]

Express your love

My patients tell me that they are titillated by knowing that they are wanted. They need their partner to be sweet to them, to give them those looks of longing, and to cherish them.

Kiss her and say: "I love you" often. Bring her flowers for no reason. Don't hide your desire for your partner. Make eye contact. Smile. Tell her that she's beautiful. Tell her that she's sexy. Touch her.

Be interested in your partner. Listen to what she has to say. Then ask questions to demonstrate that you heard her. Sometimes, when my wife is talking, I catch myself thinking about something else or thinking about what I'm going to say as soon as she stops talking. I'm working on becoming a better listener.

---

[77] Rupert Holmes. "Escape (The Piña Colada Song)" on *Partners in Crime*. Produced by Rupert Holmes and Jim Boyer. Infinity Records. 1979.

Watch for unhealthy patterns in your relationship and do something about them if there are. Is there unresolved anger or guilt? If there is, address it. Anger is not sexy!

5. MAKE SEX DATES

If you are having spontaneous sexual intimacy with your partner as often as you would like to, you can ignore this one.

For many couples—probably most—the sex becomes less and less frequent the longer they are together. When life gets in the way of regular sexual intimacy, the relationship may suffer, and the warmth and tenderness may wane.

But during sexual intimacy the brain produces oxytocin and vasopressin, hormones known to be associated with feelings of attachment. Couples can give each other a booster shot of these "love hormones" by having a sex date.[78]

Why are sex dates so powerful?

In her excellent book *Come As You Are*, Emily Nagoski describes how men and women tend to be very different when it comes to sexual desire.[79]

According to Nagoski, seventy-five percent of men experience *spontaneous desire*. This means that the majority of men want to have sex whenever they see or hear about a desirable woman or when they have a sexy thought or memory. But only 15 percent of women experience spontaneous desire. The remaining 85 percent of women experience *responsive desire* or a mixture of responsive and spontaneous desire. This means that they are not likely to want sex unless they are in a sexual situation.

---

[78] Acevedo, Aron, Fisher, Brown, "Neural Correlates of Marital Satisfaction and Well-Being: Reward, Empathy, and Affect" (*Clinical Neuropsychiatry*, Vol 9, 2012, pp. 20–31)

[79] Emily Nagoski, *Come as You Are, The Surprising New Science That Will Transform Your Sex Life.* (New York: Simon & Schuster, 2015)

The myth of spontaneous sex is that when a man is aroused all he has to do is watch for those moments when his partner seems aroused, and then make his move. Or if he doesn't see any sign of her being aroused, all he needs to do is make sexual overtures such as suggestive looks, sexual comments, or intimate touching. *Boom! Spontaneous sex!*

But if Nagoski is right and 85 percent of women seldom or never have spontaneous desire, this may explain why your sexual overtures aren't working.

What to do? The answer is to not rely on your partner being aroused but to rely on your relationship and your mutual desire to keep it romantic, sweet, and intimate.

So have a heart-to-heart talk with your partner. Tell her that you want that romance and intimacy back in your relationship. I'll bet that you will discover that she wants it too.

Make a date. Ask your partner what you can do to help take some of life's pressures off her so that she is more available to set aside some time with you for sexual intimacy. Tell her that you want to arrange time for a date to make love.

Ideally, this would be at least once a week. The weekly timing doesn't have to be rigid of course, but it might help to agree as a couple how often your dates will be. And consider renegotiating the frequency over time.

Once you and your partner are in a sexual situation, you have created exactly the setting that Nagoski tells us 85 percent of women need in order to experience responsive desire. Since you two have probably been together for a while, you already know what she responds to, so you're halfway there. And as your communication as a couple continues to improve, you can learn even more about ways to please each other.

MAN QUESTION

Get real! Are you suggesting that we schedule our sex?

DR. D's Answer

Yes, that is exactly what I'm suggesting. This concept is actually becoming de rigueur. See what *GQ* says in its May 2012 edition:[80]

It may not be a bad idea to schedule sex. Seriously. On the one hand, it sounds like the death of all that is worth living for. Scheduled sex? What's next? Scheduled smiles? But bear with us: It is easy to fall out of the habit, especially if you have kids. You get busy; you get tired. Suddenly you look up and you haven't been laid in four months. This is not good. Your brain is in danger of absorbing a dangerous idea: I can live without sex.

Sex, in addition to feeling good and keeping you from murdering people who annoy you, is good for things like intimacy with your spouse. And scheduling it is a way of making sure that intimacy doesn't get away from you.

Thanks, *GQ*. Nicely put.

BACK TO NANCY'S STORY

Everything is normal on Nancy's exam, so we sit down to talk.

"Many woman past age forty tell me that their sex drive is going or gone," I say. "The waning sex drive is partly from the drop in estrogen levels that occurs during a woman's menopausal years. But so many women have also told me that their sexuality seems to have been swept aside by a multitude of distractions in their lives.

And a woman's sexual desire is usually very different from that of a man. Most women respond better to a planned sexual situation than to a spontaneous one." We talk about spontaneous desire (usually the man) versus responsive desire (usually the woman).

Nancy remains silent, so I continue. "If you wait until you're in the mood for sex, it's not likely to happen very often, if at all. And couples who don't

---

[80] *GQ*'s Marriage Survival Guide, "You'll Want to Bang the Cleaning Lady. And That's Normal" (*GQ*, May 2012, p. 170)

have regular sex tend to become distant from each other as a result of the lack of intimacy."

I suggest to Nancy that many couples regain that intimacy by having regular sex dates. I tell Nancy more about sex dates.

When I see Nancy for follow-up a few weeks later, she seems more upbeat. "I was feeling pressured and uncomfortable when Mark approached me for sex. I was almost never in the mood. Having sex dates has taken away the awkwardness. Now that I know when we're going to make love I have time to get in the mood. And we make sure that the date is at a time when we aren't tired or distracted. Now I'm able to relax and enjoy the intimacy."

Mark has come to the visit with Nancy. He is also smiling. "Making dates to make love is working way better than I thought it would," he says. "I don't feel so compelled to constantly hassle Nancy for sex. I know that I am going to get the sex that I want instead of excuses. I have time to take a shower, shave, and brush my teeth. And I'm in less of a hurry while we're making love because it's happening on a regular basis."

Romance and sex are natural and easy at the start of a relationship. But as time passes the realities of life happen and the romance and sex may wane. Fortunately, aroused or not and erection or not, couples benefit from regular sexual intimacy.

Broken record: Romance is like a plant. No matter how hardy and beautiful it is when you get it, you have to take care of it to keep it beautiful and alive.

WHAT'S NEXT?

In the last chapter, we'll review a brief summary of concepts that I think deserve to be emphasized.

And in the appendices following Chapter 11 you will find a great deal more. In Appendix 1, I discuss the pros and cons of hormones. In Appendix 2, I cover certain hormone-free medications that are often used for menopausal symptoms. And in Appendix 3, I talk about natural remedies for menopausal symptoms.

Parting Thoughts

Menopause is a natural change that all women go through. A woman's body, her mind, and her experience of life undergo dramatic changes at this time. Usually, at about the same time, men are also going through major changes.

Our experiences of life are changing and not necessarily in the same way as our partner's. These processes and their effects raise questions that need to be answered by both partners.

- Is this the beginning of the end? Or is this the beginning of the next phase of our life together?
- Are we going to renew our commitment to each other and parlay these changes so that our relationship gets even stronger and more nourishing? Or are we going to allow these, sometimes divergent, changes to push us apart?
- What will my partner do to optimize her health and comfort during menopause? And what can I do to support her?
- What can I, the man, do to optimize my health and hygiene so that I continue to be healthy, feel good, and remain attractive to my partner?
- What can I, the man, do to keep our relationship equal and romantic?
- Our sexual relationship may have changed—or ended. We may seem to be more like roommates now. Am I—are we—willing to do what it may take to get the romance, sweetness, and tenderness back?

Here are some strategies that can address every one of these questions, issues, and concerns.

- Look at your relationship together to assure that you support and respect each other and that the power dynamics are equal.
- Recommit to each other and to a sexually intimate relationship.
- Don't ignore menopausal symptoms such as vaginal estrogen deficiency, which can result in a dry and tender vagina. Talk about them and encourage your partner to get medical help.
- The same goes for you, the man. If you are having problems getting and maintaining an erection, talk with your partner about it. I'll bet that she's way more supportive than you think. And I'll bet that she already knows.
- Go see your doctor about any issues of concern. If you don't feel comfortable talking with your doc, maybe you need to find another.
- Don't avoid sexual intimacy. Just approach it differently—with awareness, care, empathy, and planning.
- Plan sexual intimacy together, preferably at least once a week.

Menopause can be the beginning of the next chapter in the love story of your lives together!

Hormones—Doc, Give 'em Back to Her

Taking estrogen, the primary female hormone, will improve most if not all of your partner's menopausal symptoms.

MAN QUESTION

So, hormones are the way to go then, right?

DR. D'S ANSWER

Maybe, maybe not. Hormones can be used at any age to reduce the symptoms of menopause, and they are usually very effective at this. But the older a woman gets the higher are the risks of using hormones. After age sixty—and even before age sixty for some women—the risks of taking hormones for menopausal symptoms are higher than the health benefits. Your partner will want to talk with her doctor about whether hormones are right for her.

How Estrogen Is Taken

Estrogen can be taken by mouth, by skin patch, by vaginal ring, and by topical (skin) emulsions, gels, and sprays. Each approach has its pros and cons.

By Mouth

Estrogen pills are taken once or twice a day.

Pros: They're easy to take and less expensive than other methods of delivery.

Cons: They need to be taken every day. And hormone levels fluctuate, higher right after the pill is taken and lower by the time the next dose is due.

Skin Patch

Estrogen can be absorbed through the skin from a skin patch. The patch can be applied to the abdomen, back, hip, or thigh. The patch is replaced once or twice a week depending on its type.

Pros: The patches are available in multiple strengths depending on the amount of hormones needed. Estrogen levels will be more consistent with the estrogen patch than with estrogen pills.

Cons: The patches are more expensive than the estrogen pill. They can cause skin irritations. They sometimes fall off (although when they do, they can be replaced). And some women may not like the aesthetics of a skin patch on their body.

Estrogen Vaginal Ring

Femring is the vaginal estrogen ring currently used in the United States for menopausal hot flashes. It is a soft Silastic ring, which can be inserted into the vagina. It stays in place continuously and is replaced every three months. Most women don't feel it once it's in place. And men usually don't feel it during intercourse. The ring stays out of the way of the penis by tucking itself between the vaginal folds.

Pros: Once the ring is in place there's nothing to do with it for three months. The hormone levels don't fluctuate because they are continuously absorbed over the three months. The steadier hormone levels that are produced by the ring may control hot flashes better.

Estrogen is being delivered through the vaginal wall, so the ring also provides excellent maintenance of vaginal estrogen levels. As a result, the vagina will be more moist and elastic and tougher for sex.

Cons: The estrogen ring is more expensive than the estrogen pill. A woman, or her partner, needs to be comfortable inserting the ring and replacing it every three months (although it's actually easy to do). It's possible—but not likely—that the ring can be felt during intercourse. If so, it can be taken out for sex and put back in afterwards.

Estrogen Topical Emulsions, Gels, and Sprays

These liquids are applied directly to the skin on the shoulders, arms, buttocks, or thighs.

Pros: These are another option.

Cons: The gel and spray are more expensive than the estrogen pill, although the emulsion is not. Their application is more involved and it has to be applied every day.

MAN QUESTION

Is it true that my partner has to take two hormones in menopause?

DR. D'S ANSWER

That is true if your partner has not had a hysterectomy (surgical removal of the uterus). If she still has her uterus, the estrogen must be combined with a progestin (progesterone or a progesterone derivative).

Estrogen by itself will excessively stimulate her uterine lining, which could lead to abnormal bleeding or uterine cancer. The progestin will prevent this excess stimulation.[81]

HOW PROGESTIN IS TAKEN

Progestin can be taken by mouth, by skin patch, and by topical (skin) emulsions, gels and sprays. There is also a progestin intrauterine device (IUD). There is no progestin vaginal ring currently available.

By Mouth

A progestin tablet can be taken at the same time as the estrogen tablet. There are also combined estrogen and progestin tablets.

Pros and *cons* are the same as with the estrogen tablet.

---

[81] MacMahon, "Overview of Studies on Endometrial Cancer and Other Types of Cancer in Humans: Perspectives of an Epidemiologist" (*Seminars In Oncology*, Vol. 4, No. 1, Suppl. 1, 1997, pp. S1-122–S1-39)

Skin Patch

Skin patches containing both estrogen and progestin are available. *Pros* and *cons* are the same as with the estrogen patch.

Progestin Topical Emulsions, Gels, and Sprays

There currently are no Food and Drug Administration (FDA) approved progestin preparations that can be applied directly to the skin. Formulating pharmacies do offer these, but the proper dosage is not regulated or well understood.

Progestin Intrauterine Device (IUD)

Progestin IUDs are tiny plastic devices impregnated with progestin. One is inserted through the cervix into the cavity of the uterus by a doctor during an office visit. Depending on which type is used, they continuously release progestin into the uterine cavity for three or five years.

Pros: The progestin IUD has been suggested to be the best approach to providing progestin to women who are on menopausal estrogen. The advantage of the progestin IUD is that it places the progestin directly into the uterine cavity and is thereby highly effective at preventing estrogen from overstimulating the uterine lining.[82] And with minimal absorption of the progestin into the rest of the body, there are minimal side effects.

Cons: I was disappointed to read recently that the progestin IUD was associated with a 19 percent increased risk of breast cancer in a study of 94,000 Finnish women ages thirty to forty-nine.[83]

---

[82] Wildemeersch, "Potential Health Benefits of Continuous LNG-IUS Combined with Parenteral ERT for Seamless Menopausal Transition and Beyond—A Commentary Based on Clinical Experience" (*Gynecological Endocrinology*, Vol. 29, No. 6, 2013, pp. 569–73)

[83] Soini, Hurskainen, Grenman, Maanpaaj, Paavonen, and Pukkala, "Cancer Risk in Women Using the Levonorgestrel-Releasing Intrauterine System in Finland" (*Obstetrics and Gynecology*, Vol 124, No. 2, Pt. 1, 2014, pp. 292–9)

The progestin IUDs are expensive so check to see if your insurance will cover them. An office visit is required for their insertion. And the insertion may be painful.

Hot off the press! SERM instead of progestin

DUAVEE which is estrogen combined with bazedoxifene (a SERM) is now being marketed as an alternative to estrogen-progestin therapy for hot flashes. Drugs in the SERM class act like estrogen in certain parts of a woman's body and act like an estrogen antagonist in other parts. Like progestins, the SERM, bazedoxifene, inhibits estrogen from stimulating the endometrium. DUAVEE has been shown to reduce hot flashes by 75 percent.

DUAVEE appears to strengthen bone. It also appears to have no effect on the breasts, so no increased breast tenderness and no increased risk of breast cancer. As with estrogen, blood clots forming in the legs and potentially traveling to the lungs or brain are more likely with bazedoxifene.[84]

BIOIDENTICAL HORMONES

MAN QUESTION

What are bioidentical hormones?

DR. D'S ANSWER

Bioidentical hormones are the exact copies of the hormones that are naturally made by a woman's body.

Until recent years, bioidenticals could only be obtained at compounding pharmacies (drug stores, which process bulk hormones into pills, creams, and suppositories). Fortunately bioidentical hormones are

---

[84] Silverman, Christiansen, Genant, Vukicevic, Zanchetta, de Villiers, Constantine, and Chines, "Efficacy of Bazedoxifene in Reducing New Vertebral Fracture Risk in Postmenopausal Women with Osteoporosis: Results from A 3-Year, Randomized, Placebo and Active Controlled Clinical Trial" (*Journal of Bone and Mineral Research*, Vol. 23, No. 12, 2008, p. 1923)

now available by prescription in many forms. The prescription varieties are subject to FDA regulation and so are way more reliable in dose and potency.[85]

MAN QUESTION
Aren't bioidentical hormones the best way to go?
DR. D.'S ANSWER
Um, not really.

They are touted to be better and safer than the synthetic and animal-derived hormones that we were using before bioidenticals became available. But there are no reliable statistical studies that confirm bioidentical estrogen or progesterone to be one bit safer or more effective than hormones from any other source.

I prefer the bioidentical hormones that are available by prescription; it just makes good sense to me. But current evidence does not show them to be any safer.

FOLLOW-UP MAN QUESTION
Hmm. So if my partner's body naturally stops making hormones, and since there are risks to taking them, wouldn't she be better off not taking them?
DR. D'S ANSWER
Well, yes and no. Yes, the risks of hormones would be eliminated if she didn't take them. And no, she wouldn't enjoy the benefits of hormones if she didn't take them. Let's look at the benefits and risks.

BENEFITS OF TAKING HORMONES
The benefits of hormones for menopausal symptoms include:
- Fewer or no hot flashes.
- Better vaginal lubrication and more comfortable sex.

---

[85] Cirigliano, "Bioidentical Hormone Therapy: A Review of the Evidence" (*Journal of Women's Health*, Vol 16, No. 5, 2007, p. 600)

oc, Give 'em Back to Her

- Lower risk of os _____ the bones).
- Improved skin _____ less dry skin.
- Healthier teeth.
- Lower likeliho _____ and depression.
- Lower risk of c

MAN QUESTION

Wow! That sounds great. Let's get going on hormones. But wait, what about the risks?

DR. D'S ANSWER

Great question!

Yes, there are risks of potentially serious complications in women taking menopausal hormones—especially in women taking hormones for more than five years and in women past age sixty taking hormones. Since most women on menopausal hormones are younger than sixty, I'm going to go into detail about the benefits and risks of women younger than sixty who take hormones for less than five years.[86]

There is one set of risks if your partner still has her uterus. And there is a different set of risks (lower) if she has had a hysterectomy. See the following section and table for more about these risks.[87]

COMBINATION MENOPAUSAL HORMONES

Estrogen provides excellent relief of menopausal symptoms. But estrogen by itself can excessively stimulate the endometrium (uterine lining), leading to abnormal bleeding or growth patterns, or even cancer. If your partner still has her uterus, her doctor will probably recommend combination hormone therapy: two hormones, estrogen and progestin. The progestin counteracts estrogen's excess stimulation of the uterine lining.

---

[86] Santen, Allred, Ardoin, et al, "Postmenopausal Hormone Therapy: An Endocrine Society Scientific Statement" (*Journal of Clinical Endocrinology & Metabolism*, Vol. 95, No. 7, Suppl 1)

[87] Martin and Barbieri, "Menopausal Hormone Therapy: Benefits and Risks" (July 21, 2015, UpToDate, www.uptodate.com)

The data indicate that the benefits match the risks in women under sixty who are on combination hormone therapy for less than five years.

The following table provides a summary of the benefits and risks.

Benefits and Risks of Combination Hormone Therapy	
Benefits[88]	**Risks**
Type 2 diabetes:[89] 11 fewer women per 1,000 will get it.	Cholecystitis: 9.6 more women per 1,000 will get gall bladder attacks.
Mortality from all causes: 5.3 fewer deaths per 1,000.	Breast cancer: 6.8 more women per 1,000 will develop this cancer.
Fractures: 4.9 fewer women per 1,000 will get broken bones.	Thromboembolism:[90] 5 more women per 1,000 will have this complication.
Colorectal cancer: 1.2 fewer women per 1,000 will get bowel cancer.	Stroke: 1 more woman per 1,000 will suffer stroke.
Heart attacks: 0.9 fewer women per 1,000 will have heart attacks.	Total risks: 22.4 more women per 1,000 (2.24% more) will acquire one of the above health conditions as compared to women that age who are not on hormones.
Total benefits: 23.3 fewer women per 1,000 (2.33% fewer) will acquire the above health conditions as compared to women that age who are not on hormones.	

BENEFITS AND RISKS OF TAKING ESTROGEN ONLY

If your partner has had a hysterectomy, she doesn't have a uterine lining that could be overstimulated by estrogen. So she can take estrogen without the progestin.

Current studies show that the risks of taking estrogen only are lower than the risks of combination hormone therapy.

---

[88] Benefits and risks are for women under age 60 who are on combination therapy for five years or less as compared to women the same age who are not on hormones.

[89] The milder form of diabetes that usually does not require treatment with insulin shots.

[90] Blood clots that form in the legs and can break loose and travel to the lungs or brain.

Benefits and Risks of Estrogen Only	
Benefits[91]	**Risks**
Type 2 diabetes: 11 fewer women per 1,000 will get it.	Cholecystitis: 14.2 more women per 1,000 will get gall bladder attacks.
Mortality from all causes: 5 fewer deaths per 1,000.	Thromboembolism: 2 more women per 1,000 will have this complication.
Fractures: 5.9 fewer women per 1,000 will get broken bones.	Stroke: 1.2 more women per 1,000 will suffer stroke.
Heart attacks: 3.8 fewer women per 1,000 will get heart attacks.	Total risks: 17.4 more women per 1,000 (1.74% more) will acquire one of these health conditions compared to women that age who are not on hormones.
Breast cancers: 1.5 fewer women per 1,000 will develop this cancer.	
Total benefits: 27.2 fewer women per 1,000 (2.72% fewer) will have the above health conditions as compared to women that age who are not on hormones.	

MAN QUESTION

Whoa! My head is spinning! So are menopausal hormones safe or not?

DR. D'S ANSWER

Data at this time suggest that in women younger than sixty who take combination hormone therapy (estrogen plus progestin) for less than five years, the benefits are about the same as the risks. And in women younger than sixty who take estrogen only for less than five years, the benefits appear to outweigh the risks.

Doctors also consider quality of life to be a valid reason to prescribe hormones even in women who have other risk factors.

---

[91] Benefits and risks are for women under age 60 who are on five years or less of estrogen only as compared to women the same age who are not on hormones.

FOLLOW-UP MAN QUESTION

What about women who want to take hormones for more than five years? And what about women who are sixty and older?

DR. D'S ANSWER

Current studies indicate that for women who take hormones for more than five years and for women age sixty and older who take hormones, the risks are significantly higher and usually outweigh the benefits. That said, no woman is a statistic.

It is much more difficult to sort out the benefits and risks to women in this category who are taking menopausal hormones. If your partner is older than sixty or has been on menopausal hormones for more than five years, her doctor will help her decide whether to continue them.

What lowers the risks of hormone use?

- Taking hormones prior to age sixty.
- Taking hormones for less than five years.
- Taking a lower dose of hormones.
- Taking estrogen only. But this is possible only if your partner has had a hysterectomy.

What might raise the risks of hormone use?

- Cigarette smoking.
- Any health condition that is associated with an increased risk of stroke, heart attack, blood clots, or breast cancer.

LET'S REVIEW

Your partner may suffer from the symptoms of menopause after age forty when her ovaries begin to lose their ability to provide her with estrogen. Hormones are the most effective medications to relieve your partner's menopausal symptoms.

Her missing estrogen can be replaced using estrogen pills, skin patches, vaginal rings, or topical emulsions, gels, and sprays.

If your partner still has her uterus, she must also take, a second hormone, progestin, to prevent abnormal vaginal bleeding and uterine cancer. Or she can take DUAVEE which is estrogen combined with a SERM.

Depending on your partner's age, health status, and length of time on hormones, the risks of taking hormones may outweigh the benefits. Even so, her doctor may prescribe them for quality of life as long as the risks are understood.

WHAT'S NEXT?

In Appendix 2 we will discuss certain hormone-free medications that can relieve menopausal symptoms.

Using these medications avoids the risks of hormones. But they may be less effective for some women. And they have side effects and risks of their own. But women who don't tolerate hormones may do well on them especially if moodiness or anxiety is a problem for them.

Hormone-Free Medications

There are three kinds of hormone-free medications that may be helpful. Except for paroxetine, use of any of these hormone-free medications for menopausal symptoms is considered to be off-label. In other words, it's legal to use them for hot flashes, but the FDA has not officially approved them for this purpose.[92]

SSRIs FOR HOT FLASHES AND MOODINESS

Selective Serotonin Reuptake Inhibitors (SSRIs) are a group of antidepressant medicines. Some of them, such as Paxil (paroxetine), Celexa (citalopram), Effexor (venlafaxine), and Lexapro (escitalopram),[93] have been found to reduce the frequency and severity of hot flashes by as much as 60 percent. And they can be an excellent remedy for moodines.[94]

The most common side effects of SSRIs			
Drowsiness (17%)	Dizziness (11%)	Headache (10%)[95]	Blurred vision (6%)
Decreased sex drive (17%)	Insomnia (11%)	Dry mouth (7%)	Nausea (6%)
Weight gain (12%)	Anxiety (11%)	Rash or itching (6%)	Constipation (5%)

---

[92] Nelson, Vesco, Haney, Fu, Nedrow, Miller, Nicolaidis, Walker, and Humphrey, "Nonhormonal Therapies for Menopausal Hot Flashes: Systematic Review and Meta-analysis" (*Journal of the American Medical Association*, Vol. 295, No. 17, 2006, pp. 2057–71)

[93] Santen, Loprinzi, and Casper, "Menopausal Hot Flashes" (Mar 27, 2015, UpToDate, www.uptodate.com)

[94] Hirsch and Birnbaum, "Selective Serotonin Reuptake Inhibitors: Pharmacology, Administration, and Side Effects" (Oct 13, 2014, UpToDate; www.uptodate.com)

[95] Hu, Bull, Hunkeler, Ming, Lee, Fireman, and Markson, "Incidence and Duration of Side Effects and Those Rated as Bothersome with Selective Serotonin Reuptake Inhibitor Treatment for Depression: Patient Report Versus Physician Estimate" (*Journal of Clinical Psychiatry*, Vol. 65, No. 7, 2004, p. 959)

MAN QUESTION

Hmm! That's a lot of stuff. Maybe my partner should take hormones instead?

DR. D'S ANSWER

Maybe, but here's the deal. SSRIs are just one of several approaches to treating bothersome menopausal symptoms. Some women who are in menopause don't want to take hormones. And some are not able to take them because of medical problems. Yet they have hot flashes or moodiness that is quite bothersome. Many decide to try an SSRI and do fine on it. And SSRIs usually help them with their moodiness or depression.

The side effects are dose-dependent (worse with higher doses) and tend to lessen with continued use. So hopefully your partner will get the results she wants on a dose that is low enough to avoid bothersome side effects.

GABAPENTIN FOR HOT FLASHES

Gabapentin is a medication developed for the treatment of seizures and chronic pain. Clinical studies have shown that it reduces hot flashes by about 45 percent. It is best taken at bedtime because it also usually helps with sleeplessness.

The most common side effects of gabapentin[96,97,98]		
Dizziness (22%)	Eye twitching (8%)	Diarrhea (6%)
Drowsiness (20%)	Loss of coordination (7%)	Weakness (6%)
Fatigue (11%)	Tremor (7%)	Ankle swelling (5%)

[96] Gabapentin: Drug information. Copyright 1978–2014, Lexicomp, Inc. All rights reserved. www.uptodate.com.

[97] Guttuso Jr, Kurlan, McDermott , and Kieburtz, "Gabapentin's Effects on Hot Flashes in Postmenopausal Women: A Randomized Controlled Trial" (*Obstetrics and Gynecology*, Vol. 101, No. 2, 2003, p. 337)

[98] Casper and Santen, "Menopausal Hot Flashes" (Feb 14, 2011, UpToDate, www.uptodate.com)

Again, there are lots of potential side effects with gabapentin but it is another option. Some of my patients have done well on it.

CLONIDINE SKIN PATCH FOR HOT FLASHES

The clonidine skin patch is a blood pressure medication that was found to reduce hot flashes in some studies but not in others.[99]

The side effects of clonidine seemed to bother my patients more than the side effects of the SSRIs or gabapentin, so I seldom prescribed it.

LET'S REVIEW

If your partner needs medication for her menopausal symptoms but does not want to take hormones, an SSRI or gabapentin may be just the ticket for her.

The hormone-free medications can be less effective than hormones for most women, but they can make your partner's symptoms more tolerable.

There are fewer risks from taking the hormone-free medications. Each has a long list of potential side effects, but many women do well on them. The side effects are dose-dependent (worse with higher doses) and tend to be less bothersome over time.[100]

WHAT'S NEXT?

In Appendix 3 we will review the most commonly used natural remedies for menopause. We'll look at how effective they are and what side effects they produce.

---

[99] Nelson, Vesco, Haney, Fu, Nedrow, Miller, Nicolaidis, Walker, and Humphrey, "Nonhormonal Therapies for Menopausal Hot Flashes: Systematic Review and Meta-analysis" (*Journal of the American Medical Association*, Vol. 295, No. 17, 2006, pp. 2057–71)
[100] Casper and Santen, "Menopausal Hot Flashes" (Feb 14, 2011, UpToDate, www.uptodate.com)

Natural Remedies for Menopausal Symptoms

Natural remedies are appealing because they don't require seeing a traditional medical doctor or obtaining a prescription. Let's first look at herbal and nutritional remedies. Then we'll discuss alternative medicine and life style alterations.

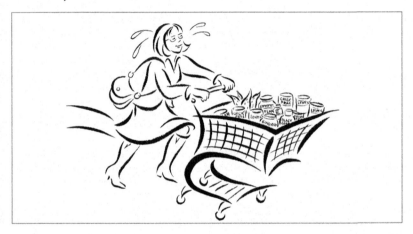

HERBAL AND NUTRITIONAL REMEDIES

These aids for menopausal symptoms can be obtained over the counter and are for the most part derived from plants. The popular notion is that they are safer than prescribed estrogen. They probably are safer because their estrogen activity is weaker. However, the FDA does not regulate herbal and nutritional remedies. This makes it difficult to verify their proper dosage, safety, and effectiveness.

Current statistical studies show that the effectiveness of herbal and nutritional remedies at reducing menopausal symptoms is questionable. But everybody is different. Some women swear by them. Your partner is not a statistic; she may find them to be helpful.

Commonly used herbal and nutritional remedies[101]		
Herb or substance	**Dosage and effectiveness**	**Cautionary notes**
Black cohosh[102] is a Chinese and Native American root-extract remedy for hot flashes and moodiness.	The usual dose is 20 to 40 mg twice a day as needed. It is one of the most widely used menopausal herbal remedies, but as yet there are no good studies that show it to be beneficial.[103]	Side effects can include nausea and vomiting, headache, and low blood pressure. Black cohosh has potential estrogen effects, so your partner should not use it if she has been advised to avoid hormones. It has been reported to be associated with liver damage in some cases.
Vitamin E is normally present in our bodies.	The usual dose is 800 units daily. Vitamin E supplementation has been shown statistically to reduce hot flashes very slightly. The benefit was minimal.[104]	Potential side effects include fatigue, headache, diarrhea, nausea, and blurred vision. Your partner should also take 65 mcg (micrograms) of vitamin K each day, because vitamin E has a potential for causing vitamin K deficiency.
Soy foods, chickpeas, and lentils	All contain a plant compound called isoflavone, which has mild estrogen activity.	A potential harm is that they may stimulate breast cancer growth, although the statistics that suggest this are very weak.[105]
Flaxseed (alpha-linolenic acid and linseed) contains the plant compound lignan.	This can be taken to improve hot flashes, but its effectiveness has not been statistically demonstrated.	Flaxseed can increase your partner's tendency to bleed from cuts and could cause temporary hypoglycemia (low blood sugar) or hypotension (low blood pressure).[106]
Red clover (trifolium pratense, beebread, cow clover, and purple clover) is an herb that is used for hot flashes.	The usual dose is 500 mg daily. Red clover contains phytoestrogens (plant extracts that have some estrogen activity).	Your partner should not use red clover if she has been advised against taking estrogen. This herb has also been associated with bleeding tendencies.
Ginseng (ninjin) is a root extract taken for hot	The usual dose is 50 mg to 300 mg twice daily. There are	Potential side effects include diarrhea, nervousness, skin rash, insomnia, breast

101 Casper and Santen, "Menopausal Hot Flashes" (Feb 14, 2011, UpToDate, www.uptodate.com)

102 Also known as actaea racemosa, black snakeroot, bugwort, and rattle weed.

103 Nedrow, Miller, Walker, Nygren, Huffman, and Nelson, "Complementary and Alternative Therapies for the Management of Menopause-related Symptoms: A Systematic Evidence Review" (*Archives of Internal Medicine*, Vol. 166, No. 14, 2006, pp. 1453–65)

104 Barton, Loprinzi, Quella, Sloan, Veeder, Egner, Fidler, Stella, Swan, Vaught, and Novotny, "Prospective Evaluation of Vitamin E for Hot Flashes in Breast Cancer Survivors" (*Journal of Clinical Oncology*, Vol. 16, No. 2, 1998, pp. 495–500)

105 Messina and Loprinzi, "Soy for Breast Cancer Survivors: A Critical Review of the Literature" (*Journal of Nutrition*, Vol. 131, Suppl. 11, 2001, pp. 3095S–108S)

106 Dodin, Lemay, Jacques, Lugar, Forest, Messe, "The Effects of Flaxseed Dietary Supplement on Lipid Profile, Bone Mineral Density, and Symptoms in Menopausal Women: A Randomized, Double-Blind, Wheat Germ Placebo-Controlled Clinical Trial" (*Journal of Clinical Endocrinology & Metabolism*, Vol. 90, No. 3, 2005, pp. 1390–7)

flashes, moodiness, fatigue, stress, and forgetfulness.	no good statistics that confirm it to be effective.	pain, and palpitations. There is also potential for high blood pressure, blood sugar fluctuations, and bleeding tendencies.
Dong quai (angelica sinensis and tang quai) is a root extract.	The usual dose is 200 mg twice daily. It is taken for fatigue and hot flashes. Its effectiveness has not been substantiated.	Possible side effects include nausea, vomiting, and diarrhea. If your partner is sensitive to estrogens, she should not use dong quai, because it is rich in phytoestrogens (estrogens naturally found in plants). Dong quai has also been associated with bleeding tendencies.
Evening primrose oil (oenothera biennis, fever plant, king's cureall, night willow-herb, and scabish) is an herbal seed extract.	The usual dose is in the range of 500 mg to 8,000 mg daily. It is used to treat depression, fatigue, breast pain, and hot flashes, but no good statistical studies confirm it to be effective.	Potential side effects include nausea, vomiting, and diarrhea. It may increase the risk of seizures, bleeding tendencies, and hypoglycemia (low blood sugar).
Wild yam (dioscorea villosa or colicroot) is a tuber (root) used to treat menopausal symptoms.	The usual dose is 250 mg one to three times a day. Its effectiveness is uncertain.	Possible side effects include nausea, vomiting, and diarrhea. Women sensitive to estrogens should not take wild yam, which is a member of the phytoestrogen family.

ALTERNATIVE MEDICINE AND LIFESTYLE ALTERATIONS

Naturopathic physicians and **homeopathic physicians** offer a variety of approaches and remedies for menopausal symptoms. They can help your partner with diet, lifestyle, and herbal treatments.

Chinese medicine, which is very different from conventional Western medicine, is an approach that has been helpful to some women.

Acupuncture is worth a try. To this date, there is no convincing statistical evidence that acupuncture is beneficial. But some women do find acupuncture helpful.

Lifestyle alterations are discussed in detail in earlier chapters. They can make a big difference in improving menopausal symptoms.

LET'S REVIEW

Some women find herbal and nutritional remedies to be very helpful at improving hot flashes, moodiness, and sleeplessness. Safety, effectiveness, and proper dosage are not well established because the FDA does not regulate these remedies.

Naturopathic physicians, homeopathic physicians, Chinese medicine physicians, and acupuncturists are often experts in natural menopausal remedies. Your partner may want to seek their professional advice.

Anything that makes your partner physically and emotionally healthier will make it a little easier for her to get through these discomforts.

About the Author

My father was a family doctor in Lafayette, Indiana. Both my older brothers followed his footsteps and went into medicine. I followed their lead and got my medical degree from Indiana University. I especially enjoyed obstetrics and gynecology as a medical student and so completed my obstetrics and gynecology specialty training at Indiana University Medical Center.

During the four decades of my obstetrics and gynecology practice, women have confided to me their most personal thoughts, insights, and concerns. I feel privileged to have had their trust.

I am now retired from practicing medicine. I love retirement. I'm busy with writing and myriad other projects. But I do miss the joy of participating in the birth of new lives, and the warmth and satisfaction of interacting with my patients and their families.

I live in Seattle, Washington, with my wife and a funny little Labradoodle. My two adult daughters, whom I adore, have moved beyond the boomerang phase and also live in Washington.

CPSIA information can be obtained
at www.ICGtesting.com
Printed in the USA
LVOW13s2204181217
560207LV00042B/2639/P